Dear Heart

Dear Heart

*Life-Saving Stories From
Women To Women*

Pamela Serure

CPW Communications
New York

Published by CPW Communications

For information about permission to reproduce selections from this book, write to CPW Communications LLC, 350 Central Park West, Suite 12G, New York, New York 10025.

An earlier version of this book, entitled *Take It to Heart*, was published in the United States in 2006 by Morgan Road Books.

This book in not intended to take the place of medical advice from a trained medical professional. Neither the publisher nor the author takes any responsibility for any possible consequences from any treatment, action, application of medicine, herb, or preparation to any person reading or following the information in this book.

Library of Congress Cataloging-in-Publication Data available upon request.

To...

The power of the heart, and to all the women
who hold that power inside themselves,

My parents Gloria and Hy, for all their love and
nourishment through this ride called my life

And to my puppy, and best heart ally, Habebe,
who on a daily basis turns my heart on.

What a heart on is:

**The place where intuition lives, the language
that comes from inside the heart, and the ultimate
"aha!" of the whole heart.**

CONTENTS

Foreword by Brenda Strong xi

CHAPTER 1. WAKE-UP CALL *1*

CHAPTER 2. THE FAMILY BUSINESS *27*

CHAPTER 3. OVER MY DEAD BODY *63*

CHAPTER 4. THE BOOK IS SEALED *93*

CHAPTER 5. THE THREE STOOGES OF HEALING:
            DISBELIEF, DENIAL, AND DEPRESSION *123*

CHAPTER 6. THE WHITE SALE: EVERYTHING MUST GO *155*

CHAPTER 7. WHERE IT STOPS, NOBODY KNOWS *173*

CHAPTER 8. WHEN LIFE GIVES YOU LEMONS *189*

*Appendix. Straight from the Heart: Resources for Women
            with Heart Disease* 207

Acknowledgments 223

FOREWORD

When I first met Pamela Serure, I had just been cast as Mary Alice Young on *Desperate Housewives*. After my untimely death, my character was to be the voice of what was going on in the hearts and minds of the women of Wisteria Lane. From my viewpoint of "somewhere in omniscient advantage," my character illuminated what was at the heart of each character. *Desperate Housewives* struck a chord that resonated with women everywhere. How well do we know what is in our neighbor's heart, and more importantly, how well do we know what's in our own?

We are at a time in history when heart disease is the number one killer of women in America. This fact begs the question, what is happening in the hearts of women? *Dear Heart* is the book every woman should read to jump-start her own heart, educate herself about the real truth about heart disease, and give her a platform to help other women. Let's be honest about what we need to transform inside and out. Why do we as women typically take care of everyone else first? This book is about caring for the physical heart and the spiritual heart as well.

Pamela Serure has written an honest, funny, and compelling journey into her own heart. Through her near death experience, Pamela discovered the truth about her own heart. In *Dear Heart* she reveals the stories that string multiple women's hearts together like Chinese lanterns lit up to illuminate the path ahead for us all. The cover touts the claim, "Telling the Truth about Women and Heart Disease," and the book doesn't disappoint. Pamela bounces back and forth between true stories that pull at your heart and hard facts that inform your head. We get the feeling that any of these stories could be us, and if we don't listen to her advice and get ourselves checked, it might be. *Dear Heart* is a cautionary tale, but not one intended to frighten so much as empower, entertain, and enlighten.

Pamela does not fit the standard heart disease patient profile. A healthy life style expert and non-smoker, this fit, fresh, raw fruit juice "foodie" shows us that the face of heart disease is as unique as a strand of DNA. Pamela's lean frame and bright smile are not what one would typically expect from someone who has advanced atherosclerosis. By educating us through the facets and faces of each story, in particular hers, we begin to get the message that it's not so important what we look like on the outside, as how we look and feel on the inside.

Heart disease touches all ages, races and socioeconomic categories of women, and is finally getting it's fair share of attention in the news. The world is changing. Women are becoming leaders not only of families and communities, but in government, law, medicine, science, and education. History is being made and women are in positions of leadership at a crucial time on our planet. The unstable world economy and the health crisis are calling us all to shift the focus from over consuming and return to an authentic balance. Historically the balance of every family is held in the arms of the mother figure. If our mothers disregard, sacrifice and overextend themselves, we learn that it's okay to disregard, sacrifice and overextend the resources of mother earth as well. The ineffective model of ignoring the whispers of the planet cannot continue, just as we cannot ignore the whispers in our own hearts. We are experiencing a spiritual wake up call.

How can we change this old model of over extending our selves and our resources? We as women can start to affect change globally at home and at work. We need to start taking care of ourselves, from the inside out. Every choice we make from what we buy to what we feed our families speaks volumes about what we value in our hearts. How we think, feel and the choices we make affect the happiness and health of our hearts, both physically and metaphorically.

Here is just one example of why the old model doesn't work.

My mother raised six children through sweat and sacrifice, love and courage, after which she took care of her own elderly mother, and gave selflessly until she suffered a massive stroke at the early age of sixty-seven. She planned to travel to see where her ancestors were from in Scotland, but her stoke took away her freedom. I watched her put others first all my life, and even though she loved us deeply, the cost was a stroke leaving her paralyzed until her death fourteen years later. Because of her love, I am motivated to change how women take care of themselves, oftentimes last.

I believe that the old model of the sacrificial mother doesn't work any longer; it is unsustainable at the very heart. As women we can give and take care of ourselves, we can teach our children to honor their feelings, by nurturing our own, we can teach compassion by accepting who we are and not comparing ourselves to the covers of magazines. This is a new age in how women relate to themselves, we are learning that to take care of others, we have to have a full well before we offer others a drink. We are learning that the way to a man's heart is through our own. We are starting to understand that we can't give when we don't receive.

We as women have given out of love and service from the beginning of time, often at the cost of our own health. Now it's time to receive out of love and service to our selves and to the health and balance of our families and the greater good of the planet. We are being called forward to embody the Divine Feminine principle. The Divine Feminine principle is one of receiving life and manifesting from authentic purpose and community. This is exactly what Pamela has done with this book. She has received a deeply affecting life experience, and by letting in the truth and import of it, she can now align herself with the purpose of helping women everywhere and impact the world community by educating them about women's heart disease. She created a non-profit organization called Events of the Heart, whose mission is to tell the story at the heart of every woman. By educating through entertainment, women are touched, motivated and inspired to make a difference. This is what happened when Pamela had the courage to tell the truth about what was going on with her own heart. Each of us has a story. We become closer through this ancient art of storytelling and our tribe gets stronger. If I've learned nothing else from my role on *Desperate Housewives*, it's how important one voice can be.

I have been working with Events of the Heart to bring the stories of women's heart disease forward through the arts. I also helped Women Heart and Metamucil to launch the Beautify your Heart program to help to educate women of their heart risk and to empower them before they have a heart attack. Giving women the key components to a healthy heart lifestyle that affect change in their lives, could save them from going through what Pamela and countless other women have. When you hear the stories of countless women who are told they are "just anxious and should go home," or "they are just imagining their symptoms and are fine" you realize there is a profound gap in equal care for women when it comes to heart health. With medical professionals telling us we are "imagining" our symptoms, when do we begin to listen to our instincts? Now.

This is a new paradigm; we as conscious educated women need to be the leaders, asking our health care providers, and ourselves some tough questions. We need to listen to our hearts, create sustainability in our own lives first, then the ripple effect will move out into our communities and into our policies and onto the planet. We are the caregivers, and care receivers, but also the keepers of the truth. We need to know our blood pressure and cholesterol numbers, know our medical family history and know what questions to ask our doctors. We need to know what turns our "*heart on*" as Pamela so aptly writes.

What would the world look like if we followed our hearts? Beautiful. And, not so "desperate" after all.

—BRENDA STRONG, Actress and Health Advocate

Creator of Strong Yoga4Women™, specializing in the field of fertility, spokesperson for The American Fertility Association, Events of the Heart, Beautify Your Heart, Metamucil, and women's wellness. Brenda is a 500hr EYRT Yoga teacher, writer and award winning actress and lives in Los Angeles, California with her husband and son.

1.

WAKE-UP CALL

I always thought of my life as a real heart-on.
That is, up until the day my heart turned off.
—Pamela Serure

This book is about a broken heart. Not the variety that comes from a disrupted family or a disillusioned love affair, nor the kind brought about by a longing that has never been fulfilled. Not that I haven't experienced those; I assure you I have endured all the varieties. But this particular story is about a different sort of heartbreak—the heartbreak caused by heart disease.

The Heart Truth

Heart disease is the #1 killer of American women.

—American Heart Association (AHA), 2005

I have always thought of my heart as being *on*—vibrant, open, optimistic, and exuberant. Ever since I was a kid, I had believed that everything was possible. I knew that I was wanted and loved by my parents and my large family, and I was raised to be all that I could be (even if I was a girl). That feeling always fueled my confidence to pursue my dreams and nothing ever stopped me. That feeling also birthed my relentless hunger to know everything I could. Being a born Scheherazade, I always enjoyed playing to the crowd, never shy or fearful, living for adventure after adventure. Fast was the speed I always operated on while slow was the one I rarely used.

I never married or had children, because somehow I got it in my head that I would be giving up the freedoms I was so desperate to gain. Looking back on those choices, I recognize the profound emotional gratification I deprived myself of. Instead of birthing babies, I chose a multitude of business and careers—designing jewelry, merchandising and creating fashion, and innovating and implementing alternative health concepts. Although these brought me recognition, accolades, and awards, I missed not having children. I missed not having someone to mentor, someone who would teach me about myself as I have watched my friends be taught by their children. But as they say, God had other plans. Even though there was a satisfaction I attained along with some hard-earned success, my definitions of success changed each decade. Many of my friends achieved a level of fame as well in those years, so playing on the fringes of celebrity was always another way to distract those maternal pangs.

In my early 40's I wrote my first book, *3 Days to Vitality*, based on my healthy detox program, Get Juiced. I had become a juice fasting guru amongst the Hampton set and was already two decades into meditation and yoga, even though I was operating on my internal mantra which was "do more—be more, have more." I binged on stress whenever and wherever it appeared. It was familial, natural, and necessary for my existence. Stress is the diet of choice for women on the fast track, and I am a born sprinter. Stress was the habit I sipped like a triple latte. But just like caffeine, stress provided only a false sense of being energized, and it barely kept me afloat. Not to mention its constant companions: cortisol, the stress hormone, which ravages the body, and adrenal fatigue, a burnout condition all of us stress junkies eventually experience. In never stopping, never taking no for an answer, never being or doing enough, I was wearing my heart out while my mind kept on going. Sound familiar?

I was at an exhilarating point in my life and I still believed that I could do anything or keep trying… up until the day my heart changed direction. That is when I had to hold up the flag of surrender to the "More" and "Go"—commands by which my life operated on. Heart disease is a shock to all who experience it, and to me it was simply surreal. I had no choice but to view it as my biggest wake-up call: I had to stop everything in order to listen to what my heart needed to live. Heart disease forced me into accepting the relentless drives and emotions I had kept in check for years: doubt, fear, judgment, and needing to be more. Those drives had kept me away from a deeper place of rest, gratitude, and trust in my life. I needed to get to that place and accept that was the only place that was going save my life.

♡ *Heart disease is the body's way of saying stop: Stop driving yourself, stop overreaching, stop trying to fix the world. Just stop whatever it is that you were so hell-bent on doing and breathe.*

All my dreams, confidence, creativity, and healthy living could not protect me from where my heart was about to take me…which was not, as I'd often hoped, to the love of my life or to all my dreams fulfilled, but to a 99% blockage of my arteries and triple bypass surgery. I had *heart disease*, the old man's disease, the how is that possible for a 47 year old meditating 110 lb women disease. Heart disease is for people who don't take care of themselves, I was obsessed with self care. The disease of denial for a yoga fit, vegetable eating, non smoking, doing all things healthy women. I was no longer feeling the glow of the Golden Child, nor like the lucky person, my grandmother said I would be, I was an alien unto myself and had nothing to turn to for reference. I had always been told I was special and I did believe it, but this leveled that belief for me in minutes. Special is when you believe nothing can penetrate your aura, special is when ordinary doesn't penetrate you, special is when the facts belong to someone else. As it turns out, I was so *not special*; I was a cookie cutter case of a woman with heart disease—the family disease, the stress disease, the *numero uno* disease for women. I was one of every three women and 1 of the 8 million now living with heart disease. I was a mere statistic.

The Heart Truth

1 out of 3 American women will die from heart disease.

—AHA, 2005

In the ten years since my first heart event, I've arduously come to terms with that journey. For starters, I had to admit to myself I had been broken hearted—from promises not kept, from love un-met, from genes unknown. Second, I had to stop. Stop all the movement, the nonsense, and above all the drama that fed my heart disease more than it could handle. I had to focus instead on attending to my heart, and savoring the little pleasures, re-prioritizing the demands, and relearning how my new life wanted to be lived. Finally, I had to break my denial that I had a disease. I had to surrender to the truth that heart disease and I were going to be lifelong partners. Domestic partners and, if I was really lucky, a soul mate.

These days heart disease has all my attention, as it should have yours. Not only do one in three American women have it, but often death is the first presenting symptom. We die from it faster because it's harder to detect in us, our symptoms are different from men's and we take longer to get care because we don't know that those symptoms are attached to women's heart disease (and neither do a lot of doctors who are diagnosing women). Just like all the other difference between men and women the symptoms and the ways we deal with them differ greatly. Women don't want to admit to having pains and uneasy feelings, in our backs, necks, and shoulders, pains that we cant quite explain, pains that don't seem that important. Heaven forbid we should complain. In truth, heart disease is more of a woman's fate than it is a man's. *Heart disease among women shouldn't be a secret, and I am not keeping it anymore.*

Many years ago, a famous psychic told me that my destiny in this lifetime was to teach women. Of all the things I'd imagined becoming in my life and had worked to accomplish, teacher was never one of them. And yet here I am, called now to teach some truths about women and heart disease. My destiny came in an unexpected way, but it's my destiny nonetheless. I'm writing this story now because I have to; I have no choice but to follow where my heart wants to go. Because written in every woman's heart is the story of her life.

Heart Song

CATHY A., *Phoenix, Arizona*

I had my first heart attack at thirty-nine. It was just a hair-like tertiary artery, so I basically ignored it. I told myself it was no big deal. Then at forty-two, I had a massive heart attack. I flatlined thirteen times in two and a half hours. No one in Georgia had ever seen anything like it before. All my major arteries went at once.

The night of my massive heart attack was April 12, 1998. I should've been smarter. I should've known better. I'd not only suffered one heart attack already, but I was a rehab nurse at the hospital, so I worked with heart attack and stroke patients all the time. But all I did that night when I started having chest pains was call my mom. I didn't do anything else until 1:30 a.m. on Wednesday when the big pains hit and I started sweating from places I didn't know it was possible to sweat from. That's when I finally went to the hospital.

You know how sometimes you're watching a movie and it fades to black? I was sitting on the gurney, and

I did that. Last thing I thought before I flatlined was, "I'm screwed." I knew I was dead. There's no way I could hurt the way I hurt and survive. I was panicking. I was telling the nurses I work with, people who know me, "I'm dying! I'm dying! I'm dying!" They kept saying, "Calm down." I said, "I'm dead." Then I was gone, down for the count. It was a horrific situation. Every time I came back I'd start talking like I was having normal conversation, but then I'd flatline again. After six or seven times they usually let you go. But my friend Darlene who was working on me said, "She's fighting, so we have to fight, too." I was lucky to be at a hospital where the nurses were my friends. So the doctors kept going.

When I woke up seventeen hours later in the ICU I thought I was dead. I heard a funny noise and wondered why it was so dark. I thought, "What? I didn't make it to Heaven?" I could feel my consciousness trying to wrap itself around the trauma. But then as the fog began to fade I started thinking, "Wow, I'm alive?" I was amazed, as were all the nurses.

I put 99 percent of the blame for my heart disease squarely on my shoulders. I spent many years smoking, starting when I was seventeen. Even when I had that minor heart attack at thirty-nine I only quit for a year, and then I started smoking again. I was also a heavy pot smoker. I drank a lot. I was overweight. I didn't exercise other than to get up to go to the fridge. I didn't have enough respect for myself to pay attention to the gravity of cardiovascular disease. I knew all about heart disease because I worked with people who had it. Yet still I'd say, "I'll drink and smoke 'til the day I die." And I was true to my word because I did die, but I was resurrected. The doctors said, "We don't know why you're here." I said, "You know you're in trouble when you go to heaven thirteen times and they put up a sign that says, 'Do not disturb.' You know God's got some greater mission for you to accomplish in life."

Since I woke up from my heart surgery that day, I've taken my medicine, changed my diet, quit smoking and drinking, and started exercising. I was horrified to know that I had really killed myself.

But I still had battles to fight in this war. After the triple bypass, I did well for about two months and then I started having trouble again. I'd hurt real bad with angina when I lay down at night, and it would wake me up in the morning. I told my doctors,

"Something is wrong." But you know I'm afraid that when male doctors in particular see a woman coming in time and again for the same problems they say, "Oh you're just having anxiety. You're making it up." I kept saying, "Bull, you really need to listen to me."

Let me tell you something that I find incredible so that women who read this will never, ever let their doctors dismiss them again. On the Friday night before my third heart attack, I told the doctor that I wasn't feeling well. He kept me overnight on an IV feed. On June 11, the following day, another doctor came in and said, "I really haven't read your case file because it's too thick and I don't have time, but I don't see anything indicating that you're having heart problems." I'd thrown up, which is a classic symptom for women. I had a headache. But he said, "I don't see anything. I really think we've got a case of hypochondria here. I'm sending you home." I said, "Something is wrong." He said, "I don't see anything that indicates that." When the nurse came in to disconnect me from the IV she said, "The doctor wrote an order for you to go home. If you don't leave, your insurance won't pay for it." So I left. I was furious. I said, "I'll be back."

The very next day, June 12, I told my husband to take me to the hospital. I was really hurting. I couldn't manage with the sublingual nitroglycerin. As soon as the doctor ran the EKG he was barking orders like an army sergeant. The doctor from the day before walked in and started screaming about how I was a hypochondriac and got sent home. But the ER doc said, "Come look at this." He showed him my EKG. Then they both started calling for a cardiac ambulance to take me to a bigger hospital. When I got there, they said, "Gee, we're sorry, but you've had another heart attack." All that first doctor had to do was keep me in the hospital for another twenty-four hours of observation, but he dismissed me because I was a woman. He thought I was being stupid or over-reacting, so he sent me home.

My husband and I were furious. My body was going to do what it did, and I take responsibility for my heart disease. But when that doctor dismissed me, I was off the charts angry. Arrogant doctors think they know more about us than we do! When I got back to that hospital, I said to the doctor who'd told me I was a hypochondriac, "You're fired."

Luckily, God still wanted me around. I survived

my third heart attack and more. In December of 1998, I lost one of the arteries they bypassed and was on the edge of a fourth heart attack. The doctors put a stent in, then another. They said, "You're going to continue to have cardiac episodes like this until your heart stops. We don't believe you'll live another year." They sent me to a psychiatrist to help me deal with dying. I said, "Are you God? I don't need help dying! I've already done that a couple of times. I need help living." I told him to leave. God didn't put me through all this in order to die, I knew that much.

In March 1999, I started chelation. I'd been consuming one hundred milligrams of nitroglycerin sublingually per week and I couldn't walk to the bathroom without hurting. But after a year of chelation and a regimen of omega-3 fatty acids, vitamin E, and co-enzyme Q10, I wasn't even taking nitroglycerin. I was cleaning my house, vacuuming, sweeping, and taking showers without fear of keeling over. I even got a part time job. I'm fifty years old now and I plan on sticking around for a long time to come.

I have to take responsibility for the fact that I have these heart problems because of my own behavior. But I have two children, lots of friends, and lots of things I want to do. And I don't want to go yet. So I had to find a way to love myself, to fight to stay here. That meant accepting certain things: No, you don't drink, you don't get high, and you don't smoke because you like breathing a whole lot more. I had to empower myself to live. This is my choice, my destiny. *Choice* is the word. It's your choice. Some people tell me that sounds hard. Well, how much harder is it to leave your kids behind?

The thing for me is now I don't have bad days, ever. I had a bad day. It killed me. When I woke up, I understood what God was telling me about a good day. You've got this moment only. Every morning when I wake up and I'm still on this earth, it is a good day. It is an absolutely great day. Anything that happens in between, that's just a thing. I don't holler, I don't scream. I used to get all upset because I have that type AAA personality. Now when someone honks a horn I say, "Love you, too. Peace." I don't worry about any of the small stuff. I invest in myself, and if I do that then I'm investing in everyone I love and adore. You have to entitle yourself, give yourself permission to live a good life.

I go around to schools now and give talks to kids

about my experience. I tell them, "Here's what I learned. The dope dealer wasn't at the hospital, the guy at the liquor store wasn't at the hospital, and Phillip Morris didn't send a rep to say hi. You're just money to them. It's an interesting thing. I can laugh at it now." They say, "How can you?" I say, "Why not laugh? I'm not mad at them, and I'm not mad at me. I just wanted to learn and to live. And I did."

Not only did my bypass surgery open the passages to my heart; it opened my eyes. For it was then I learned that heart disease was my silent enemy, killing more American women than all the cancers combined. And yet I also discovered that most women have no idea that heart disease is their number one killer. Nor that the symptoms of heart problems in women often differ completely from the chest-clutching, Hollywood version of a heart attack. Nor that many women today are struggling to recover from their heart events by putting on a brave face in spite of their depression, shock, and shame. As women, we're amazing, strong, and nurturing. How else to ensure our legacy but to become proactive and take on heart disease as our biggest challenge?

The Heart Truth

**Only 13% of American women view heart disease
as a health threat.**

There are reasons many medical professionals discount heart disease in women, one is that for such a long time it has been taken hostage by men. Men, whose symptoms are clear and who get checked regularly for heart problems. Men, who benefit from having had many medical studies conducted on them alone. Men, for whom heart attack rates have declined in the past years while they've risen in women! Men who simply have to say "I don't feel well" and get the EKG. As a result, women are coming into hospitals complaining of shortness of breath, a burning sensation in their chests, back, neck and jaw pain, and are being told we're suffering from anxiety or stress, and sent home—sometimes *even during a heart attack*. We do receive improper treatment and inaccurate diagnoses day after day, time after time, woman after woman, and we're dying because of it. It's the shocking fact that needs a makeover.

I didn't know any of this until I had my open-heart surgery. I had never heard about it, read about it or even eavesdropped on a woman having a conversation about it.

Was heart disease the real closeted disease women never talked about? I remember when cancer was the hushed conversation across the dinner table. Mothers and grandmothers whispering who had it and keeping it quiet, as if that would make it go away. Now cancer is a constant conversation at America's dinner tables. Even after cutting me open, it took me a while to break my denial. What did I do to cause this, was this my fault? How could I ever teach health again, who would believe me? I sure didn't. When I realized the truth, coupled with the numbers, I felt compelled to make communicating these facts about heart disease my service call.

While I am aware that I'm imparting these warnings in a somewhat alarming and high-pitched manner, I must say that a heart event is traumatic and warrants the attention. Like all traumas, there always is a pearl which is born from the grinding of the soul. For me, I've found heart disease to be a tremendous source of bonding with my inner voices and internal dialogue. While it is insidious, I believe we can choose to see this disease as something that can serve to help women everywhere turn their hearts ON. Second, I've discovered that women with heart disease typically become ferocious advocates once they begin to recover. We fight for ourselves and others because we recognize that it is truly our birthright to be happy, healthy, and get the care we need and deserve. Finally, there is a component of heart disease that allows us to take a more intimate look at ourselves. For me, heart disease has served as a pathway to appreciating my inner life and myself more deeply, with a new compassion and sweeter joy. It has set a more humane pace by which I can live. It has become an antenna I use for making life choices.

♡ *When we live life according to the heart's dictates, we're both mesmerized by the fluidity of surrender and terrified by the loss of control.*

The thing is, even if you don't have heart disease now, someone close to you does or will soon: your sister, your best friend, your mother, your colleague. It's a fact of our modern lifestyle. Dealing with or preventing it is not just about reducing your fat intake or getting more exercise, as everything on the topic suggests. We also need to concern ourselves with gaining real knowledge about all the complicating factors, including family history, the way we metabolize stress, and our responses to disappointment and anger. Mine was a combo, layered like the deli sandwiches renowned in New York, a towering compilation of stress and genes. I called it The Bypass. These, it turns out, were and still are the most influential relatives in my life.

We cannot go deaf, dumb, and blind to heart disease because it's intimidating, frightening, and pervasive. The numbers are still growing, and more women are having heart attacks at young ages. The only way to shrink the numbers is by building awareness of the disease, identifying the symptoms, getting regular check-ups, and making better choices about exercising and eating right. The heart is the organ of courage and love. It is the organ of poetry and passion. Being heart savvy is the best face-lift in town—not to mention the longest lasting.

> ## *The Heart Truth*
>
> **Heart disease kills more women than all the cancers combined. Yes, including breast cancer.**

With this book, I seek to galvanize a ministry of women who will, with their wisdom and their own heartfelt stories, help me spread the word about heart disease among their networks of friends and families. I also hope to address many of your questions about heart disease. What is the personality of the disease? What are some of the many and varied symptoms? What's it like to have it? What are the most talked about remedies, treatments, and medicines? How do we live with it? How do we care for it, sleep, eat, and make love when we have it? How do we become closer to its roots in women?

♡ *If it happened to me, then it could happen to you.*

That font of emotion, the deepest, most mystical and magical part of us, the heart is the dwelling place of our true self. We know we need it to express all that we are, all that we feel, but many times we can't or don't or won't. We keep things secret that fester inside our hearts. Secrets, like plaque, harden and often leave us poised for any enemy to make the body its home. The heart welcomes joy but also carries its opposite, despair. Love has the biggest piece of real estate in our hearts, but sometimes love can go years without expressing itself. Ever wonder why we want to get things "off our chests" when we are in danger of losing someone or ourselves?

Dear Heart will serve as both recipe and remedy—a cautionary tale for women who are fortunate enough to have healthy hearts, and a source of comfort and support for the more than one-third of American women who are dealing with the disease in their lives right now or finding out each day that they have it. This book will not censor facts or feelings, although it's neither a political statement nor a blame game. Rather, this is a story from one woman to another, the only kind that spreads. I share what I've learned on my journey: what I had to change, what new and enduring truths I needed to incorporate into my life. The tool that served me best in my healing, that gave me the stamina I needed to travel this difficult road, was my humor. I peppered my pain with anything that brought laughter. I hope that you will take some time with this book, and let both the facts and feelings, fill up the place that is your broken heart, and your whole heart. I hope it empowers you to regard yourself as your highest priority and live life to the fullest.

While my personal journey serves as the backbone of *Dear Heart*, I've asked women of all ages, shapes and sizes to share the stories they carry, and they have answered soulfully, truthfully, and most important, willingly. You'll find their Heart Songs sprinkled throughout the book. I've also asked cutting-edge doctors in the field today to enlighten us as to the different faces and phases of this disease, from symptoms and diagnosis to prevention and recovery.

In order to prevent, live with, and even embrace the reality of heart disease, we must learn to move to the sound of our individual heartbeats. We must pick our battles lest they be our last. We must say what we feel in real time in case there is no more time later. We must challenge our responses instead of going with typical reactions. We must stop and consider instead of constantly plunging forward and controlling. We must give our minds a rest so that our hearts can become more alive. We must appreciate that the little moments often are the biggest ones. We must discover how to be true to ourselves and love whomever and whatever we love no matter who agrees with us.

♡ *Your purpose is your life, and your life is on purpose when you cheat death.*

As Heart Women, we have a deeper mission. When we begin our journey, we realize it is indeed a rich expedition into the mysteries of ourselves and the desires that rule us. We need to tread softly through the waters that become our tears and recognize the real sunshine in the end. I say for myself that my heart chose to turn *off* so that I could find out how to turn it *on*. *Dear Heart* is my way of living from my heart on out to yours.

Heart Song

JUDY K., *Phoenix, Arizona*

My mother died of a heart attack less than twelve hours after she was sent home from the ER. She shouldn't have died that night. She was the victim of a problem that unfortunately is far too common: Doctors ignoring symptoms of heart attacks in women.

My mother was sixty-three when she died, but she looked ten years younger. She was also in incredible shape. A week before, we'd gone walking together and she'd had more energy than I did at twenty-nine.

The day my mom died she'd been out in the sun. It was a hot day. She started feeling unwell, so she went home to rest. When she still didn't feel better a few hours later, my aunt suggested they visit an urgent care clinic near the house.

At the clinic, my mother complained to the physician's assistant assigned to treat her of tightness in her chest and jaw, pain radiating in her left arm, clamminess, sweatiness, and shortness of breath—all classic signs of a heart attack in a woman. But it was 4:45 in the afternoon on a Sunday, and I suspect the doctor just wanted to get home. He told my mother she was dehydrated from the heat. He prescribed ibuprofen, one of the worst things you can give to someone having a heart attack. (Unlike aspirin, which prevents the clots that cause heart attacks from forming and is considered one of the most important medicines for heart disease, ibuprofen may actually increase the risk of heart attack and block aspirin from working.) Then he told my mother to go home, eat a Popsicle to cool off, drink lots of water, and get some rest.

Tragically, my mother took the PA's advice. She went to bed early, complaining that she still felt ill. My grandma, who was in her late eighties at the time, found her daughter the next morning dead in her bed.

I wish my aunt had taken my mother to the hospital instead of to a clinic. I wish my mother had seen a doctor and not just a physician's assistant. I wish the PA had listened to her. I wish that one of the family members with her at the time had known more about women and heart disease. But sadly for us, this is the way things happened, a chain of errors. And my mother, a vibrant, beautiful woman, passed away as a result.

Since then, I've learned a lot about women and heart disease. Every day in the US, it's like one plane full of women crashes into the ground and dies from it. Given our family history, my sister and I are now getting our hearts checked regularly.

But the main message I have to share with other women is this: Stand up for yourself and take action. If you think there's even a remote chance that you're having a heart attack, insist on having a full set of tests. Don't worry that your family or the doctors will think you're silly if you're wrong. Take the time to get yourself checked out. If you aren't completely satisfied, ask to speak to a second physician.

You have to take responsibility for your own care. It's worth your time and money if it means that you're going to be alive the next day. My mother was not alive the next day, and I miss her.

HEART ON

QUIZ: Are YOU at Risk for Heart Disease?

PHYSICAL FACTORS

- Are you overweight?
- Do you carry most of your excess weight in the stomach region?
- Do you eat processed and/or fast food more than twice a week? Have you been doing so for years, perhaps your entire life?
- Are potatoes, carrots, and other sugary vegetables your primary sources of vegetable matter?
- Do you have high blood pressure?
- Do you have high cholesterol levels?
- Do you sweat heavily during or after the slightest physical exertion?
- Do you often have gastric trouble, reflux, or heartburn?
- Are you diabetic?
- Do you smoke? Have you ever smoked for more than a year?
- Do you have a family history of heart disease?
- Are you in menopause, post-menopausal, or perimenopausal?
- Do you take hormones?

- Do you ever experience pain in the jaw, neck or shoulder region that is unexplained?
- Are you an emotional eater who prefers fatty foods?

EMOTIONAL FACTORS

- Have you been hiding something in your life for a long time?
- Have you had more than four unsuccessful love affairs/relationships?
- Do you have blue moods more than three times a week?
- Does something feel incomplete inside you no matter what you do?
- Do you dislike your body?
- Do you admonish yourself for most of your actions?
- Do you often feel anxious, angry, or sad—or all three?
- Have you been depressed for more than three years?
- Is loneliness a factor in your life?
- Have you been heart broken more than twice?
- Do you have fits of unexplained anger or rage?
- Do you feel as though your life hasn't turned out the way you wanted and expected it to?

MENTAL FACTORS

- Do you feel as though you're never satisfied?
- Do you drive your body too hard?
- Do you need to be in control?

- Do you fly off the handle easily?
- Do you over-think each situation?
- Is everything you do wrought with stress?
- Do you feel as though there's never enough time?
- Do you have an "off" button inside yourself that you can't seem to find?
- Do you worry endlessly about everything?
- Do you have a sense of futility about the future?

If you answered "yes" to four or more of these questions, it's time to get into a conversation about what's going on with your heart. Please visit your doctor for a heart check-up exam.

2.

OVER MY DEAD BODY

The body we have, with its aches and pleasures,
is what we need to be fully human, awake and alive.

—PEMA CHODRON

How do I really pop this book open, the book about one of the most significant passages of my life? Should I simply allow the words to flow out and breathe on their own, like the vapors from a just-corked bottle of peppery Syrah? Should I pry them out like sardines folded tightly into each other in their briny placenta? Or should I be witty to help assuage the feelings inside?

I think I will begin simply by telling you that I am a woman—the same as you in many ways, but of course not exactly the same. As women, we know that we already have shorthand with one another, so I will start from there. We know what life feels like inside our bodies, how it all works when it works and how it feels when it doesn't. We know that sensation in our throats right before we want to scream, and that slow burn in our eyes when we're holding back our tears. We know how to sneak forbidden treats like lifelong thieves, and how to fain perfect innocence upon their disappearance. We know every inch of our naked bodies and still see the flaws above the perfections. We know verses of excuses and chapters on forgiveness. We just know.

♡ *For women with heart issues, honesty really comes to the forefront. It's as if clearing the plaque out of your arteries also rids you of the lies inside. There is a fear, with heart issues looming, that any day might be your last. What if you didn't tell the truth? Whom would you betray in the end?*

Women are a code as much as we are a gender. So it really doesn't matter if I tell you that my hair is short or long, dark or light, if my eyes are blue or green or brown. It shouldn't matter if I tell you that I lost five pounds on the Atkins diet, or that I like dark chocolate more than milk. I would still be the same as you are or were or will be, sometime or somewhere in your life.

If we were all in a room together, we would probably first check each other out in a superficial way, making passing judgments about each others' clothes, hair, makeup, body firmness, plastic surgery—the full checklist. But then, as time wore on, we would progress to revealing the deeper wounds from our mothers, our lovers, and all the small tragedies we hold so deep within us—the wounds of our hearts, the scars of our souls. Yet no matter the differences, we would bond in the end, sipping wine, laughing, and probably eating a delicious feast someone had prepared. Because when women gather together we know how to nourish each other with our wisdom, compassion, and humor. We would end our time with a dessert or two to remind us that tomorrow always holds a sweeter promise.

If we sat long enough in that room together, we would certainly notice that we are, as women, more the same then we are different, including the fact that most of us either have heart disease, will have it, or know someone dear to us who has it. I am just one of voices in the chorus of that room.

The Heart Truth

Every minute, a woman dies from heart disease.

—AHA, 2005

Heart Song

FAYE R., *Manhattan, New York*

Aghast, dumbfounded, horrified…and then I fell into a state of shock….On February 10, 2003, at the age of twenty-eight, I was told I'd had a stroke. The above were just a few the emotions that engulfed me after having an MRI and being told the news.

My life had been spent living very healthfully. I was an athlete and active my entire existence. I enjoyed eating healthfully and had a busy and fulfilling life in New York City. I had just started a public relations business the year prior to my stroke. Of course, I had heard of a stroke, but in my mind that was something that only afflicted the elderly.

February 9, 2003 was a unique morning. I was woken up at 4:00 a.m. by what I call "brain pain," pain like nothing I'd ever experienced in my life. When I got up I was dizzy and had trouble seeing, all of which I blamed on being groggy. I took an aspirin to alleviate the pain, but after an hour it had not abated. I was in acute pain and I tried taking another type of aspirin hoping that would work. By 9:00 a.m. I decided to reach out to my doctor, but the receptionist said that they could not see me until the following week. Something told me that I needed to see a doctor right away, so I became more insistent with the receptionist.

I arrived at the doctor that afternoon and told him my symptoms. He explained that I'd had an ocular migraine and prescribed a migraine medication. At the same time, he advised that I visit with my eye doctor because of the vision interruption I'd been experiencing. Somehow I managed to get myself to the eye doctor, ambling down Third Avenue with limited vision. Once I was there, I was asked to take a vision test where I saw green dots that blinked. I thought I was going crazy, and after five minutes I explained I could no longer do the test. Obviously, I had failed miserably. The eye doctor suggested that I go to a neurologist. Back out on the street, I got myself to the neurologist who prescribed an MRI and at that point, I had nothing left in me. I went home and needed to be in bed. The following morning I went to the MRI center (little did I know they can see a stroke in an MRI). When

I got off the table and got out of the room, there was a group of doctors waiting for me and they asked me to pick up the telephone. It was my neurologist who said that I'd had a stroke and needed to head over to Lenox Hill, where he'd meet me.

Once at the hospital and under close supervision, I found out that a blood clot had lodged into the ocular section of my brain cutting off blood supply and causing vision impairment. The pain was largely from the swelling in that area which is how they can detect a stroke on an MRI. I saw the images of my brain with a white mark in each of them…that was the damage from the stroke.

Today, I am very fortunate. I do still have vision impairment, but it's moderate and my brain has acclimated and adjusted remarkably well. But there isn't a day that goes by that I take my health for granted. I wake up each day and I am grateful. I listen to my body very closely, and am aware of how I feel and whether or not I should take action. In the meantime it's my mission to make anyone around me aware of the signs of heart disease and stroke, the no 1 and 3 leading causes of death in our country.

I always believed that I would be the first to know intuitively if something were *really* wrong with me. After all, I often say that the greatest tool a woman possesses is her intuition. But now I make an addendum to that proclamation: Intuition only works if you want it to work. Not knowing is sometimes easier than knowing. But the more I muffled my voices, the louder they became. What you resist really does persist.

The Heart Truth

Sixty-four percent of women who die suddenly of cardiovascular disease had no previous symptoms or awareness that they even had the disease.

—AHA, 2005

In my forty-sixth year, I made an impromptu move from Manhattan and the Hamptons for a self-mandated time-off period. Something inside me knew I just needed to go where I had never been before, a place where I could be new to myself and a place that offered me some rest. LA seemed to fit the bill.

I wasn't sure if something was wrong with me; but I knew that I was not quite right. It was more than malaise and not quite an illness (which I was accustomed to after a lifetime of getting and conquering obscure maladies such as shingles and scarlet fever). And yet after six months in LA, I still didn't feel well. How could I be "not right" after having moved so far way from home, into the sunshine overlooking the shores of Malibu? How could I be "not right" in a place where every morning I could peer out over the idyllic dolphin-strewn playground called the Pacific? How could I be "not right" with the farmers' markets on a daily basis beckoning, feeding my addictions to fresh fruits, flowers, and breads? How could I be not right when time was all I had now? How was that possible?

♡ *Denial is the internal prosecutor for emotions not ready to be revealed. Denial can make one believe that which is unbelievable.*

My nagging symptoms felt like walking pneumonia (something I'd had many times before), except for the fact that there was this persistent burning in my chest, like heartburn without eating the garlic, and a pain in my neck, and exhaustion that didn't dissipate no matter how much I rested. I knew this could be due in part to my daily visits from the Goddess Estrogen, infamous for her spontaneous mood swings, tumultuous hot flashes, and fierce heartbeats. My feeling was that if all the women in the world could synchronize our hot flashes, we would truly give new meaning to the term *global warming*. But at forty-seven, wasn't I a bit young for this harsh a version of the passage?

I think it's safe to say that most women always have some symptoms that warrant a check-up. But stress and exhaustion simply have become the modern way of life for us, like having to lose those five extra pounds no matter what the scale says. We're warriors, never thinking about a way or time when we won't feel too tired, too stressed, too put upon. So instead of setting an appointment, we self-diagnose and self-medicate, relying on time-tested remedies like chocolate, facials, cosmos, and massages. If that doesn't work, we finally, reluctantly resort to that doctor's visit.

Heart Song

TERESA R.

I had a heart attack in late July 2006. I was thirty-eight years old. I was a successful businesswoman, who worked long hours in a stressful job. I had been feeling fatigued for several months, but I blamed it on my job. In July 2006, I was cleaning my house and preparing for a weekend visit from family when I began feeling like I was having a bad case of indigestion. Having a history of stomach problems, I just shrugged it off and kept going. I entertained my guests over the weekend including cooking, touring antique malls, and playing ping-pong despite felling progressively worse. I blamed my lack of energy on the fact that I wasn't eating a lot because of my "indigestion."

The following Monday when the guests I almost passing out after taking a shower. I called the doctor and got an appointment for the next day. Fortunately for me, my new doctor, whom I had never seen before, immediately thought that my problem could be my heart instead of my stomach. She believed this in part because of my family history of heart disease. She did an EKG and saw that my heart was in distress. I was told that I had a heart attack sometime in the days prior.

Over the next week, I had two angioplasties and received five heart stents. One artery was one hundred percent blocked and the other was ninety-five percent blocked. Fortunately, I was truly blessed and I had no damage to my heart, even after waiting for such a long time to get treatment. I was stunned to be a thirty-eight year old with heart disease. I just didn't really believe that women had heart disease that young. My life has totally changed since I had my heart attack. I went back to work for one year. Then I decided that my stressful job wasn't worth the damage that I was sure it was causing to my health.

So, I quit. My husband and I moved back to his hometown in Kentucky, the town where we met and got married more than a decade before.

In addition to a stressful job, I was overweight, had a terrible diet, and didn't exercise. After the heart attack, I lost sixty pounds, converted to a totally heart healthy diet, and began exercising six days a week. The weight has been off for almost two years now. I also became an advocate for the American Heart Association and have contacted my legislators many times trying to encourage them to pass laws to assist with heart disease and health care.

I would advise all women to know what the symptoms of heart disease are and never assume that you are too young to have this chronic illness. Keep in mind that women's symptoms are different from men's and aren't what you see on a TV show. Also don't ignore your body when something doesn't seem right. Go to the doctor and get it checked out. In some ways I have been blessed (which may sounds odd to say) because this disease has caused me to re-evaluate what is important and taught me to take the time to experience many things that I never would have before my heart attack.

What was my body trying to tell me anyway? Most likely it was a call to slow down after having just completed a worldwide book tour and a move from East to West. Ya think? But to me, admitting that I was exhausted at this point in my life was not an option because what would follow that? I had no second act lined up yet. It felt far too vulnerable to stop now. It felt like I was failing at being me, betraying my own mantra. And after years of defending my life and the way I chose to live it, that would have been the white flag of surrender. It wasn't time yet for that, or so I thought. In truth, the white flag had already raised itself; I had no choice in the matter. I was too tired to keep denying it.

The Heart Truth
BY DR. JESSE HANLEY

Just as we all have different ways of laughing and crying, so too are our symptoms—the ways in which illnesses make themselves known to us in our bodies— different. But one thing is certain: When the arteries carrying blood in and out of the heart are blocked for a while, you will feel tired. Very tired. *Life* tired.

Women are used to living in this exhausted state, so it's even more urgent that we become hyper-alert to the particular signs of heart disease. We need to know the difference between a bad hair day, PMS, a fight with our significant other, five extra holiday pounds… and the beginning of a disease that now is being tracked in women as young as thirty.

When illness is present, our appetites—for food, sex, fun, energy—all seem to diminish. Depression, stomach and gastric disturbances, restlessness, anxiety, pains in the back, jaw or neck, and a burning in the chest are some of the key signs of heart disease in women. Women also frequently experience a sense of hopelessness that starts to pervade the spirit. Depression seems like a familiar friend that just moves in to stay for a while and then stays for good. Please, pay attention to these signs. Don't just write them off as the everyday side effects of stress. They could be your *wake-up call*. They could save your life.

So in time, I caved in. I couldn't ignore this "not-right" feeling any longer; I had to see a doctor. At least I found a great one. Dr. Jesse Hanley is a renowned specialist on menopause—perfect for my condition. She came out to greet me wearing cowboy boots and a pink and turquoise almost-mini skirt. Wow, LA never disappoints! As I barreled through my list of ailments, Dr. Jesse was totally absorbed. It was as if I were a storyteller and she were waiting for a particular ending. The visit was magical. She was real, she listened, and she spoke in a language designated for women's ears—soft, direct, smart, and caring. She was a women's doctor for sure.

Dr. Jesse instantly picked up that I was an energy junkie feeding my habit daily with stress cocktails. She officially welcomed me to the Adrenal Burnout Club, which is what people who run on stress for too long inevitably join at some point in their lives. Forget type A, she said I had the perfect AAA personality required for membership. She introduced me to the idea of naps, saying they would change my life. I smiled at the novelty and simplicity of the idea. New Yorkers don't take naps; we have another latte. She also told me I was in perimenopause and gave me a complete list of remedies, herbs, vitamins, and protocols to deal with that.

But then she did something I hadn't anticipated. She insisted that I have my heart checked. When I questioned her recommendation, she said it was just a feeling she had about me, since my father had some valve and blood pressure issues. "Let's check your heart." I'd never heard that before. But I wasn't concerned. Doctors like to check things out; it's part of the ritual. I told her I'd do the test in a few weeks, after I got back from a trip home to NYC.

The Heart Truth

**Certain diagnostic tests and procedures for heart disease
are not as accurate in women as in men, so some
physicians may avoid using them. These doctors may
not detect heart disease in women until later,
resulting in an increased risk of heart attack or stroke—
and with more serious consequences.**

—AHA, 2005

There is never a good time to hear about your impending death, especially when you feel it is untimely. The human being would rather imagine, fantasize, or create the scene than succumb to it. Yet hardly ever is it the way we envisioned. On a daily basis, just like birth announcements, news of death is delivered in the oddest ways. Mine was announced on an ordinary, sunny Southern California day at the end of September 1998.

♡ *Illness is a fantastic lens. It offers perspective and foresight
at the same time—the ultimate snapshot of a life.*

I'd taken the CT heart test that Dr. Jesse had ordered shortly after returning to LA from NYC because chest pains were now on my list of ailments. So after the test, I got home and planted myself in the womb of my new bedroom. I was gazing inward, thinking about this enormous move I'd made from

New York to LA, from cold to hot, from crazy to calm, from me to not me. I was thinking about my cocker spaniel, Sage, and how she wouldn't let me walk up the hills of Malibu with her. Day after day, she would tug on the leash till I would eventually give up and come home. Sage was a sage indeed. I was just sitting there when providence entered along with the sea breezes.

The phone rang. On the third ring, I picked up. "Ms. Serure?" the voice asked. The tone instantly set off alarms.

"Yes?"

"The results of your CT scan are terrible," came the voice on the other end of the line. "In fact, they're life threatening. I've never seen a score this high on a woman your age with your profile. Your calcium score is like dairy cow in Wisconsin and you could have a heart attack walking across the room." I collapsed inside myself and went deaf to the rest of the conversation. My unlived life circled me as ferociously as the tornado in *The Wizard of Oz*. A heart attack! I had never remotely considered the possibility of a heart attack. I mean I'd thought of cancer of course, pneumonia always, even an exotic island disease, but never ever once, not even in a drama queen moment or a passionate writing frenzy, did heart attack occur to me. Here I was with time off in paradise, and hell was my gatekeeper. There was no way that I knew of to process this kind of information, and so my only release was to burst out crying.

Within the next hour, Dr. Jesse showed up at my house, visibly shaken. Given the CT scan results, she convinced me to see a cardiologist that was part of the network she belonged to in LA. *As soon as possible.*

♡ *You always know when something big is knocking. Whether you choose to answer the door or not, it will find its way in if it belongs to you.*

Two days later, I sat impatiently in a burgundy tufted leather sofa in the cardiologist's office. I stared with glazed-over eyes at the dark green walls checkered with lack-luster oil paintings of mallards and cocker spaniels. Ralph Lauren wanna be decor in sunny LA? What was I doing here, really? I thought of the thousands of remedies I'd swallowed over the years, my commitment to exercise, and my strict organic diet. I recalled the hundreds of hours spent in ashrams, doing yoga, chanting, and meditating to ensure my sanity in stressful situations exactly like these. And yet here I was, at only forty-seven. Could I really have heart disease?

Finally I was called into the doctor's office, and a-testing we went: echocardiogram, fine; EKG, fine; heartbeat, fine. All systems normal... So what gives? I knew I was right. I always like to be right, but in this case especially. I didn't have heart disease. It was clear to me that something else was going on. Something no one had ever seen before. The doctor gave me his standard apologetic speech—better to be safe than sorry, blah, blah, blah. I excused myself to go to the ladies' room and let out a huge sigh of relief.

But like a cue coming from backstage, that persistent burning in my chest reappeared. It wasn't until that precise moment that I actually felt appreciative of being in a doctor's office. He could uncover the source of my symptoms right then and there. Instant gratification—how appealing to a true New Yorker.

I marched back into the doctor's office and said, "*Now*. Test me now. I have that burning sensation I was telling you about." For the fist time in the visit the doctor stirred, moving out of his Doctor Zone. He repeated what I'd just said about "this burning sensation thing" back to me three times, in three different ways.

"You have it now?" he asked.

"Yes, test me now while I have it!"

"You have it just walking to the ladies' room and back?" he asked again, a bit more emphatically this time.

"Yes!" I replied. Why was this so difficult for him to understand?

"Just walking across the hall?" (No, I'd joined Cirque du Soleil in the interim.)

"Yes, yes, and yes!" I replied.

"Ms. Serure," he said, looking as serious as an actor playing the doctor part on TV, "I'm afraid we can't let you leave this office."

"What?"

"This burning sensation means that you have unstable angina and you could have a heart attack just from walking across the room. So I can't let you leave my office."

"What?" I repeated, panic creeping into my voice.

"We must admit you to the hospital immediately," said the doctor. "You could die at any moment."

Hospitalization? Die? Now? "I can't do this!" I shouted. "I have to go home. I have to walk Sage. I have to get my toothbrush. I need my cashmere blankie."

"I'm sorry, that's not going to happen," he said as he placed a wheelchair before me. "We need to get you in *right now*."

"I swear I'll come back later," I pleaded (meaning later, like after getting three other opinions, later, though I did not say that out loud). But apparently my acting and negotiating skills, like my energy levels, were waning, because I was having zero effect.

Within the next five minutes, I was ushered at the speed of the opening minutes of an *ER* episode into St. John's Hospital, a destination a long way from home. Along the ride in, faces melted into walls, morphing like computer images, and the sounds and smells became psychedelic. If you've ever had the experience where it takes forever to get admitted into a hospital, watch what happens when the staff hears the words "heart attack" and sees a thin, healthy-looking woman in her forties being wheeled in… Within the time it takes to order a Big Mac and fries, I was hooked up to monitors recording all my bodily functions, bedpan included.

The Heart Truth

More women than men die of heart disease each year, yet women get only thirty-three percent of the total angioplasties, stent procedures, and bypass surgeries, twenty-eight percent of the implantable defibrillators, and thirty-five percent of the open-heart surgeries.

—WOMENHEART, 2005

Hours later, I was in an operating room being prepped for an angiogram. A multitude of doctors began their procession into the room, muttering under their breath while assuming their positions. The thumping of my over-stimulated heart grew louder and louder with each passing minute. The characters were all suited up and moving around like background dancers in a music video. They gave me five milligrams of Valium, and then they began. They cut a small pinhole in my groin and snaked a wire with a tiny camera lens through me to capture the images of my heart. Kinky! Next, they shot me full of hot liquid chemicals. A warming sensation spread underneath my skin, like taking a nuclear pee. These chemicals provided the doctors with the knowledge they needed in the colors that mattered to find out what was *really* going on.

Suddenly, there we were—the doctors, the nurses and me as a collective—staring at my tie-dyed heart, my broken heart, my exhausted, overworked heart, holding on for dear life. When I saw that image on the screen above me, it was apparent to me that this was all true: My heart had me held captive.

Abruptly, a big man leaned over and whispered in my ear. "Ms. Serure," he said in a hushed tone, as if it were a seduction, "Ms. Serure, I'm John Robertson, Chief of Cardiac Surgery here at St. John's. We're all marveling at your condition." Thank God, I thought, an intervention in all this drama, someone finally bearing good news. No such luck. "I have some bad news and need to give you some time to process this."

Wasn't the news bad enough already? Was I being *Punk'd*?

Finally, this anonymous doctor was seeing me as I have always seen myself: An urban mystic in the flesh. Never give up on being discovered; you just never know when it'll happen! My inner drama queen felt crowned and nothing could ever compete with the coronation. Nevertheless, this was not exactly how I'd pictured my coming out party.

"I am going to give you two days to get your family here and your affairs in order. We don't know if you have even two days to live, but I know you will need that time to integrate this information. You need an immediate triple bypass, open-heart surgery. Your main artery is 99 percent clogged and two other arteries are 75 percent clogged. We don't understand how you've been managing even to walk around much less fly on a plane without having a heart attack so far. You must have some great relationship with God because frankly, there is really no explanation as to how you haven't had a fatal heart attack."

Two days to sum up a life, a legacy, a destiny? My affairs

could take at least a year to put in order. At least the doctors and I agreed on one thing: I was nowhere near the typical profile of a heart patient. This was to be my ultimate betrayal—the betrayal of being all things healthy. The betrayal of thinking "healthy living" supersedes stress and genetic predisposition. And believe me, betrayal by your own belief system and your own body is much worse than any a lover could ever deliver. This had to be wrong. Whose karma had gotten mixed up with mine?

But no matter how hard I tried to deny it, on that redundant sunny California day I finally had to concede that the battle had turned into a war, whether I liked it or not. Heart disease had invaded my body, unfriendly and uninvited. What choice did I have but to enter the ring with my dukes up, ready for the fight of my life? Round one was about to begin.

HEALING THE HEART

Signs and Symptoms of Heart Disease in Women

BY JESSE HANLEY, M.D., author of *Tired of Being Tired*, co-author of *What Your Doctor May Not Tell You About Premenopause*

When Pamela Serure first came to see me, she had diagnosed herself—a New Yorker trait, no doubt. She wanted me to confirm her premature entry into menopause. But her symptoms and her diagnosis did not match—not even close.

It was not in my medical literacy to expect heart disease in such a young, vibrant, non-smoking, thin, healthy woman still having a normal menses, so I did not set out looking for that. But over the course of our appointment, I noticed a few clues as to what was really going on.

As I carefully took down Pamela's medical history, she revealed several important facts: A family history of heart and vascular disease, and a diet heavy in carbohydrates. Even though the carbs Pamela ate were supposedly the best kind (fresh raw fruit juices), the fact is that she had been living on sugar and adrenal (stress) hormones for years—a dangerous cocktail for the heart according to modern medicine.

Nor did Pamela's labs and menstrual history reveal menopause. In fact, her symptoms of fatigue and neck pain were suspiciously similar to those for heart disease. Unfortunately, there are no clear-cut symptoms of heart disease in women in general. The classic one—shortness of breath, especially with exertion—can be insidious. Many women and doctors overlook it. Many women even ignore chest pain and simply slow down, as Pamela had been doing.

So I sent Pamela to have an Ultrafast CT scan to test for heart disease, although this was before the test was fashionable. Thank heavens I did. It was more sensitive than the subsequent treadmill test the cardiologist gave her, and we may never have recognized the severity of her case without it. I still see the Ultrafast CT scan as the best screening test, far more accurate than the standard EKG. Best of all, it is noninvasive. Fortunately it rapidly is gaining recognition and acceptance.

When the results came back, Pamela's diagnosis of advanced atherosclerosis surprised me as much as it surprised her and all who know her. Good thing my intuition was working that day and that I was paying attention, because Pamela's case served as an excellent lesson for me. Women, after all, are at least as vulnerable as men to heart disease, and given how masked their symptoms can be—as Pamela's were—doctors must review their cases with a heightened sense of importance.

Even though heart disease is the number one killer of women, the truth is yet to be revealed to us in a way that enlists all of our attention. I am a firm believer that we, the medical community, along with heart disease survivors like Pamela, must find new ways to educate and inspire women to be conscious of everything our hearts are saying. Pamela and I are great friends now, and we consider ourselves warriors on the path towards enlightening women as to the risks, symptoms, and cures of heart disease. Please, pay attention to the signs of heart disease and be an advocate for yourself.

CHECK IT OUT
The Top Five Tests for Heart Disease
BY JANE FARHI, M.D.

1. Thallium stress test: nuclear imaging test that shows how well blood is flowing to the heart muscle, usually done post-exercise on treadmill (hence "stress" test).

2. Ultrafast CT scan: particular type of cardiac tomography that provides cross-sectional images of the chest, including the heart and large blood vessels.

3. Stress echocardiogram: ultrasound test given during exercise, which visualizes the heart's pumping action and may reveal lack of blood flow not apparent in other tests.

4. Perfusion MRI: magnetic resonance imaging uses magnets to look inside the body, resulting in 3-D computer-generated pictures of the heart and large vessels.

5. Angiogram (most invasive): small catheter inserted into artery up to heart through arm or groin. Then patient injected with radiographic substance. Tiny x-ray

---

> instrument on catheter shows high-contrast images of arteries.
>
> Be informed. Be proactive. Do something good for yourself. If you're at risk for heart disease, or exhibit any symptoms, please ask for these tests.

HEART ON

My Meetings with God

I have always believed in God. I have always believed something or someone was watching over me, guiding me, and doing for me what I could not do for myself. Not everything that came my way went as planned. Whose life does? And yet still I recognized that God was present in all my actions, whether I had full appreciation for the outcomes or not.

I've taken many meetings in my life for many different reasons, but the meetings I have taken with God were by far the most important. The first occurred when I was about five years old. I'd been suffering from horrible nightmares. They were probably the garden-variety boogey man type, but at the time they seemed devastating. My parents took me to a Rabbi. He told me in all seriousness and with due authority to merely rub my forehead when I had a bad dream and God would make it disappear. Then he prayed over me and sent me on my way. Miraculously, his suggestion worked time and again.

As often happens, the older I got, the more I imagined that I was in charge and the less time I dedicated to my meetings with God. So when my heart event came around, not only did I need a meeting, I needed emergency make-up sessions. The night before the operation I had probably never been closer to God other than the day I was born. To the best of my recollections, this is how I started the meeting: "Dear God, how could I be here? Did I not listen to something I was supposed to listen to? I am so confused about what I believe in right now, God, including you! You have given me so much, so many gifts and so many possible roads to travel. I know that I have abused my energies to achieve success. I know that my priorities and my focus weren't always in tandem with you. I know that we have not communicated steadily for a while. I have forsaken a place with you in lieu of a place I thought I wanted more, outside in the world. But it is apparent here and now that I stand with you, and always have and need more than ever.

"As only you know, I might not make it through this journey you have put before me. But if you do decide to keep me, please know I wanted to fall madly in love and produce my greatest works. I wanted to be more benevolent to more people and take better care of myself. I wanted to take time to understand and appreciate my life and give thanks for that. But I need more than these two days. Please, God, I need your guidance, your grace, and your faith in me now. Thy will be done."

Even though in my childlike fearful place I felt like heart disease was punishment, my heart told me it was a soul call. For most of my life, I'd sought out the newsworthy and sometimes neglected the normal everyday stuff. That's the funny thing about being driven: you can lose the direction of your dreams and in turn they can also lose you. And in the end, losing one's dreams is really losing one's life. Those initial months following my open-heart surgery brought me right back into my relationship with my spiritual nature. I felt myself growing closer and closer to God, magnetized to the vibration of love. Finally understanding and integrating for myself the true meaning of surrender.

Naked in my fear, in my belief, in God's grace, eloquent and poetic prayers spontaneously flowed from me each day. I felt like the poet Rumi in his time of grief. What emerged from my heart event was a part of me that completely allowed my intuition to guide me, and a willingness for my mind to obey, not the other way around. Life does get a bit twisted when goals seem to be the prize. Almost dying brought me back to the proverbial realization that my *life* was the real prize. Today, my relationship with God is a partnership that cannot be undone and a meeting that can never be cancelled.

♡ *Ten thousand steps a day and ten thousand meetings with God will keep your heart healthy and alive.*

Heart Song

ALICE B., *Manhattan, New York*

I'm just twenty-eight years old. So when I say, "I had heart surgery," people say, "No way! Where's your scar?"

I grew up in Hawaii. I was something of a bookworm, but also fit, healthy and always outdoors doing stuff. I weighed just one hundred pounds. Why would I ever possibly worry about heart disease?

When I was sixteen, I was talking on the phone with one of my friends, and at some point we were laughing. I remember laughing in a certain way where I inhaled and my heart started racing. I kept talking. I felt light headed and weird, but I wasn't worried. I thought maybe I was just excited. I didn't say anything about it to anyone; I just went to bed. When I woke up the next morning I felt fine. I thought it was an anomaly. But then it started happening more often. My heart would just start going as if I'd run five miles. There was no way I could stop it. I'd go to bed, and the next morning it'd be gone. And yet it became more and more disconcerting.

Eventually I told my mom. One day she said she could see my shirt moving because my heart was going so hard, so she took me to the ER. The doctors weren't sure what was going on. They thought maybe it was some kind of arrhythmia. I was nervous. They tried running all these tests and gave me a heart monitor to wear in school, but still they said, "We don't know." And after a while, it didn't come back anymore so I kind of forgot about it.

Then sometime during my freshman year at Stanford, the heart pounding started up again. I would just go to sleep whenever it happened. One day it got really bad so I went to the ER. Again, the doctors ran a whole bunch of tests. They told me, "You have super ventricular tachycardia." Then one doctor brought in some med students and asked them, "This is Alice. She's 18 and she's got tachycardia. What should we do?" And they said, "Give her adenosine." "What's adenosine?" I asked. "It's a drug that'll stop this heart pounding." So they did. I felt a rush of heat run through me as if someone had constricted my heart in a medieval torture device. It didn't work. So they said, "Up it to twelve ccs." I said, "Oh my god, you're going to do it again." And they did. The pain was horrible, but it worked. They observed me for an hour and let me go.

I went back to the ER about four more times after that for the same thing. The doctors put me on beta-blockers, saying that would help. But they had to keep upping my dosage because the meds weren't working. Finally they said, "You can have surgery. That'll take care of this problem once and for all."

The idea of surgery totally freaked me out. But I talked to my parents and did a lot of research. I found out that my doctor was one of the first ever to do this surgery back in the 70's so I thought, "He can't mess it up." I also discovered that I only had a one percent chance of death. It was surgery or medication for the rest of my life, so I said, "Let's try to make this work."

Lucky for me, the surgery went really well. The doctors told me to take it easy for a while, but then I should be okay to do anything. And they were right. My heart problems went away. At first, I would be nervous when I laughed, but soon I discovered that I really *could* do anything. Nothing has happened with my heart since. Everything is fine. Every once in a while I'll feel like my heart is about to go nuts, but nothing happens. I actually think the whole experience was kind of cool and neat, kind of crazy. These days I try to stay healthy, get plenty of exercise, eat well, and take care of myself.

The doctors still don't know what caused my heart problem. I may have been born with it, or it may have developed over time. It may have been genetic or maybe something happened when I hit puberty and my hormones went into overdrive. Who knows?

These days I do a lot of volunteer work through the Miss America organization. I try to spread the word that heart disease is the number one killer of women. I tell women, "You never know when it's going to happen to you. The best you can do is to live a healthy lifestyle and go to the doctor regularly to get your heart checked. Also, be really aware of your family history." I go to the doctor every year and get a full physical done. It's tough, a tricky disease. You have to watch out for yourself.

HEALING THE HEART

The Woman's Disease

By ALEXANDRA LANSKY, M.D., cardiologist, Associate Professor at Columbia University School of Medicine, Director of the Women's Cardiovascular Health Initiative at the Cardiovascular Research Foundation

It was Christmas Eve. Sally was sitting down to dinner with her husband and her two boys, aged six and seven. She apologized that she wasn't feeling well. She had been running around all day getting the house and dinner ready for the holiday. Sally sat in silence for a while trying to ignore what was going on in her body, but the pain in her stomach and mid-chest area kept getting worse. Her husband noticed that she couldn't catch her breath and asked, "Sally, what's wrong?" She said she had no idea. So John put Sally and the children into the car and managed to get them to the emergency room before Sally collapsed.

I was the intern on call that Christmas Eve. When Sally arrived at the ER, she was having a massive heart attack. She was only thirty-six years old, a gorgeous, active tennis player and the mother of two beautiful children. Her family couldn't believe what was happening to her, nor could I. They stood there in stunned silence as I and the other doctors started compressing Sally's chest right there on the pavement of the parking lot, desperate to get her heart beating again. Thankfully, we did. I lost track of Sally after she was transferred to another hospital, but I heard that she went on to receive a heart transplant. I like to believe that she is among us today, enjoying her children, now grown.

Heart disease is devastating, and yet few women are aware of the threat it presents to them. The number of women's lives claimed by heart disease continues to rise each year in the face of a steady decline in the disease witnessed in men. Heart disease remains the single leading cause of death among women, and more women than men in the US die of it. Heart disease is your greatest health risk. This is a fact. Friends, sisters, mothers, daughters, and wives this disease will unavoidably affect you, your life and your family.

Unfortunately, heart disease is greatly stigmatized for women. As a result it does not receive the attention it deserves either from women or from the medical community—and with tragic consequences. Women delay seeking medical treatment, delays that could mean the difference between life and death. Potent preventive and therapeutic alternatives have proven beneficial to women, yet women are frequently excluded from clinical trials and doctors often fail to apply these practices to women.

Doctors commonly misdiagnose and under-treat women with heart disease even when they present with classic symptoms. One of my patients experienced progressively worse neck and jaw pain whenever she climbed stairs. She had seen a dentist, two dental surgeons, and undergone two molar extractions before coming into my office. These doctors should have noted sooner that the root cause of her pain was actually heart disease and not the need for a root canal. Another patient of mine with heart disease was hospitalized and treated repeatedly for asthma, even though she did not respond to the customary asthma treatment.

The preconceived notion that women are somehow "protected" from cardiovascular disease is simply wrong. A woman older than fifty-five years with high cholesterol, high blood pressure, and a family history of heart disease is at risk and should be under active management. The presence of diabetes, regardless of age, is a stronger risk factor for women than for men and warrants very aggressive preventive care. Approximately $200 billion is spent each year on cardiovascular health, with only six cents of every dollar spent on prevention. Spending more on educating, studying, and treating younger women now would be a wise investment in the future.

All of these factors explain why *Dear Heart* is such an important and timely book. As a female cardiologist, raising awareness about the dangers of heart disease in women, advocating more research and better treatment for women, and reducing the numbers of women who die from this disease are my passions. I feel incredibly fortunate to have crossed paths with Pamela Serure, whose energy and work is inspirational.

Ultimately, my goals and Pamela's are one and the same. We are striving to improve women's health and wellbeing today and for generations to come, so that never again will two young boys have to witness the premature death of their mother from this preventable disease.

3.

THE FAMILY BUSINESS

In women everything is heart, even the head.

—J.P. RICHTER

Nothing in life ever slips past me unnoticed. That's just the way I am. And yet I was missing the link that had brought me to this place, this operation, this unbelievable predicament I could not escape. I could not explain my life to myself anymore. Nothing I'd ever read in magazines or seen on TV or discussed with doctors or heard from my party lines of friends had ever remotely prepared or even hinted to me that what I'd been suffering from could possibly be heart disease. In fact my friends and I comprised a medical dictionary of issues and ailments. We knew every healer and everything that needed to be healed on the planet. We were the wounded generation and healing was our journey. But never in any workshop, circle, or ceremony had we healed a woman with heart disease. How could that be? In my mind, the dots did not connect.

The doctors concluded that stress and bad genes were the Gemini twins responsible for my condition. *Heart disease is a family disease*, they told me, from the blood pool your genes jump out of to the way your emotions are metabolized. And the more we looked, the more evidence we found that my family is riddled with heart disease. Only I was the biggest casualty of the bunch.

The Heart Truth

If someone in your family has heart disease, make sure your doctors know this and give you the proper tests and attention.

—AHA, 2005

Still, it was difficult at first for me to accept this explanation that I had the family disease. I mean, I knew that everyone on my father's side of the family had died from some sort of heart condition, but they'd seemed so old while I was so young. Also, they certainly didn't take care of themselves as well or have the same level of self-awareness as I did. My father had his valve replaced, but his lungs were so ravaged from years of smoking that he was predestined to suffer some consequences. I'd quit smoking when he'd gotten sick, and that was years ago. And yes, my mother had soaring cholesterol levels, but she kept on ticking and never had a problem with her heart except for years of uneventful angina. In fact, she had more energy than all of us combined.

I honestly believed that my years of healthy alternative living had bought me a reprieve from the gene pool. Plus doesn't being the black sheep of the family undo some of the genes that bind? But it turned out that my family was in my blood. There was no escaping it.

♡ *No matter who you are, what you have, what you want, or what you do, it all boils down to where you come from in the end.*

Heart Song

GLORIA G., *Honolulu, Hawaii*

At age fifty-four, I'd been swimming over a mile per day for the past six years. But then I got sick in October of 2003, so for a while I wasn't doing any exercise. When I got over my cold, I thought that I should start swimming again, but I just didn't feel like it. I didn't have the energy. And my skin was looking grey. But I thought these were just normal consequences of getting older.

Then on June 30, 2004, my business partner and I were at the airport waiting to go to Kauai to visit some clients when I started to feel overwhelmed with exhaustion. My arms felt tired and I broke into a cold sweat. I didn't feel seriously ill, but I did think maybe I shouldn't get on the plane. Now I am usually not the kind of person who lets feeling a little sick get in the way of work. So when I said I was hesitating about taking the trip, my colleague agreed that I should go home. As I walked across the airport lobby to get a cab, my briefcase felt so heavy that I had to carry it like a baby, cradled in both my arms.

On my way home in the cab, I called my husband to tell him what was going on, and I started to cry. I never cry, so I thought that was strange. Back home, I immediately took my blood pressure because I've had problems with it ever since I was young, but it was normal. I had no headache or vision problems, but I still felt awful. When my husband got home he said, "I made you a doctor's appointment for 4:30 p.m." I said, "I need to go to the hospital now." So off we went.

As we walked into the door of the ER, I said, "I think I'm having a heart attack." I don't know why, I just had this gut sense and some awareness of heart disease from reading the news. The receptionist sent me into a room and it was ten minutes before I saw anyone. The nurse took my BP, which was still normal, as were all my vital signs. Next the doctor came in to examine me. She said, "We're *sure* you're not having a heart attack, but we're going to do an EKG to rule it out."

So out went the doctor and in came the tech. The moment he put the leads on, his eyes popped out of his head. I said, "What's the diagnosis?" He said, "I'm not allowed to diagnose you, but you're having a massive heart attack right now." He started screaming for the doctor, and a bunch of folks came running into the room. Suddenly, the whole ER was in there with me. They asked me who my cardiologist was, and I said I didn't even have one. By the time one arrived, all my vital signs were going crazy. The cardiologist said the reason my BP had been normal was that I'd been in shock.

The doctors pulled someone off the angiogram table and put me there instead. It turned out that of my four main arteries, one was one hundred percent blocked, two were ninety-five percent blocked, and one was ninety percent blocked. So I was walking around with my heart getting almost no oxygen. Probably the only reason I hadn't dropped dead was because I'd been swimming and my heart was so strong.

I ended up having a quadruple bypass that very day. There I'd been, standing in line to get on an airplane at five of noon, and by 7:30 that night I was out of surgery. My doctor said that if I'd gotten on that airplane, I'd be dead. If I hadn't come into the ER, I'd be dead. The only thing he said I should've done differently was called an ambulance instead of having my husband drive me to the hospital. So from now, I won't hesitate a minute to call an ambulance for my friends or myself.

I got out of the hospital five days later. And you know what? I ended up having a wonderful summer—one of the best of my life—because everybody, all my family that lives here in Hawaii, all my friends, camped out at my house. And everyone was there to take care of me. They'd bring dinner up and we'd all eat together. It was such a pleasure. Everyone was so connected, so present. It was a magical time.

Since then, I've stopped eating cheese, which was my favorite food. I've started walking, and now I walk twenty-five miles a week. I want to get back to swimming, but I'm not supposed to do that for another four months because it takes so long for the sternum to heal from open-heart surgery. Sometimes my chest still hurts, and it's been more than a year. I take my meds and watch my weight, though I need to lose about fifteen pounds. I also get my heart tested regularly. So do all my friends and family because of me.

I don't regret at all what happened. On the contrary, I'm very grateful for the experiences my heart event brought me. Understanding your heart is really, really important. I was a little overweight, but my heart disease was mostly due to genetics and stress. So now I really have to manage my stress. I'm back at work full time, but I've started a new business and it's not so stressful.

I really want you women to know that you can't escape your genes. Your heart is your heart, and you are who you are. But that having been said, your family history isn't always as obvious as you might think. The heart disease in my mom's family was in her brother and all his kids but not my mom herself. So I never considered it genetic. You really have to expand your idea of where your genes come from. I never thought heart disease would get to me. But

I have lots of people in my life who love me, a big extended family including grandchildren, and that's what matters most.

I come from a clan of Sephardic Jews; I call us the Armani Jews because of our endless joy in celebrating and dressing up. We are a community that shows up for one another and loves to give to one another. You could say we are a family of 1,000,000. We are very traditional, religious, and sometimes borderline superstitious. We do everything in groups: three hundred strong at a Sunday barbecue, a thousand and counting at a funeral, forty plus at a holiday dinner. My clan also gives new meaning to the terms *lack of boundaries* and *co-dependency*. But they are also *always* there in numbers in a pinch. We are the original reality TV show, but then perhaps one could say that about all families. Ours is the one in Jewish Technicolor.

But there are disadvantages to growing up so closely knitted. And in my clan, the primary one is constant scrutiny—a ticker tape that runs 24/7 indicating the high-points and sell points of all whom they encounter. Everyone where I grew up knows everyone else's business. Provocative comments about people's lives spice our conversations like the cumin and cinnamon used in our delicacies. One is not only judged by who you are as an individual but by who your parents and grandparents are, how much money you have, how you've decorated your house, how you serve your guests, and who your kids marry. If you don't make waves, you can remain a part of everything until you die, and when you do everyone will show up at your funeral and speak wonderful tomes about you. But in this community, if you make waves, they become a tsunami. I adore my family and community with all my heart, but boy, have we given each other some angina over the years.

As I said, I was considered the black sheep of the family. Rather than settling down a block from my parents, marrying, and having kids as I was expected to do, I chose to move away and become a career woman. Where I grew up, "career" wasn't on the list of female life options. "She doesn't want to get married?" was both a question and a way of implying that my parents had done something wrong in rearing me. But I just knew deep in my gut that I could not live the life mapped out so clearly for me by my clan. I had to get out before it was too late. I would suffocate living next door to everyone I knew, never meeting a stranger in the course of a day, only being thought of as somebody's mother or someone's wife. I had to leave because I never would have made it any other way. And so I made waves by living out of wedlock, living in the city, and then traveling through Europe, starting my own businesses, dancing to my own tune. I always thought it was just too much for my family to handle. But now it seems it was really too much for me to handle.

♡ *The word NO has a body chemistry linking women with their heart disease.*

As a result, family gatherings sometimes became claustrophobic experiences. My dramatic life was always the focus when I returned home for a visit and it was intense. Who would react to what? I never knew. What bomb would I set off when all the family members were in attendance? What mess would I leave behind for my parents to clean up after I was gone? As it turned out, too many to count.

Not living out the story of the clan breaks many hearts: The grandmother blames the mother, the mother blames the daughter, and so it goes. The pull between being part of the clan and being separate from it was enormous, and they let me know how they felt as many times and in as many ways as they could. Who needs genes? Guilt, which causes stress, which causes plaque to build up in the arteries, was yet another connection between my illness and me.

The Heart Truth

Stress can play a bigger role in the development of heart disease than butter.

—DR. JESSE HANLEY

In later years, I learned to bring home my successes home like others brought home their grandchildren: I won the De-Beers award for jewelry design at age twenty-four; I'd opened three gift stores by the time I turned twenty-eight; I was in magazines; I was on TV, I was a designer, I was this, I was that. Yet it was hard to keep up with my brothers' children and the other grandchildren and cousins as they grew up and started talking. They were real and tangible, and a legacy my family counted on. So I'd whip out stories from my quasi-celebrity life, peppering the climaxes with tidbits from Farrah Fawcett, Barbara Streisand, Cher, Christie Brinkley, and Donna Karan. The family ate these up like the sweet date cookies and rosewater pudding my gramma prepared for dessert, making them forget what a shame it was that I wasn't married and hadn't chosen the life they'd chosen for me. Sometimes I could forget, too. I knew the secret was to leave them wanting more.

Today, I like to ask women I meet, "What happened at the dinner table growing up?" That's because the dinner table is the place where most families define themselves, and hence where the stories of who we are get played out. This is where we most learn our emotional patterns and get physically as well as psychologically nourished… or not. Chances are your family roots grow thicker than you'd ever imagined. We are impacted not just by the genetic factors but also by the everyday habits we grew up with, particularly at the table—whether they be drinking, smoking, overeating, gambling, criticizing, maligning, ignoring, laughing, supporting, sharing, or loving.

These patterns are a part of the fabric that weave a personality, mine being an oriental rug filled with colors and odd shapes. We cannot escape where we come from, no matter what geographic or cosmetic make-overs we attempt to give ourselves. Instead, we need to realize that only by exploring and understanding our family roots, following them into the deepest places inside ourselves, and accepting who we are as a result, can we trace a map of our lives. You can change and overcome many of things, but it is by blood and blood alone that lives are saved and lives are lost.

♡ *Forgive all you can—especially yourself.*

I bought my mother a gift once, many years ago, a pillow that had sewn into it the words, "Mirror, mirror, on the wall, I am my mother after all." But only after my heart event could I fully accept that and embrace it as the truth.

Heart Song

GLORIA SERURE, *Pamela's Mother*
Long Branch, New Jersey

I called my home the Movers and Shakers house. That's what life felt like with all the excitement and drama provided by me, my husband, and our two kids, Teddy and Pamela. Pamela, my first-born, was an energizer bunny. She was vibrant, funny, animated, charming, and personable. She only stopped if we sat on her or if she fell ill or went to sleep. She had enormous curiosity about everything, and she was racing to experience it all. Fast and faster were her only two speeds. In addition, she had an independent spirit. By the time she was eighteen she was living on her own, which wasn't done in our community. But Pamela had her own ideas about how she would live her life.

The sixties, seventies, and eighties were a remarkable career time for Pamela. Getting married and having a family wasn't what called her. She manifested her ideas into successful products and grew businesses. Even when she was exhausted, her indomitable spirit didn't let her stop. I often asked, "Pamela, when are you going to catch up to your physical being?"

Eventually, she did reach a place where she no longer wanted to live in Manhattan and work as a marketing executive. So she moved to the Hamptons and began exploring an alternative healthy lifestyle. That lifestyle became the inspiration to create a juice business. Get Juiced was the talk of the town. Suddenly Pamela was leading juice retreats to Bali and had a bestselling book. But with all the concentration she devoted to health for others, she neglected her own.

After Pamela finished a worldwide book tour with endless TV and radio interviews, I finally saw her low battery light flashing for the first time. Reality had set in, but we had no idea what was coming.

No parent could or should ever be prepared for what happened next. It was Jewish holiday time and as usual the whole family got together to celebrate. Pamela had just moved to LA a few months prior but came home to New York to spend a few days with us. We were thrilled. Her whole trip home she complained of burning in her chest and diagnosed herself with pneumonia. Now almost every year of her life she would get sick on these holidays, so I must admit I was a little deaf to it. I did, however, eventually take her to meet with my husband's doctor, a heart and lung specialist, even though we much would've rather been shopping, talking, and running around having fun.

After taking an hour of our precious little time together, the doctor appeared and said, "Pamela is experiencing *angina*." We—in complete unison for the first time in our lives—said, "That's impossible!" He wanted her to check into the hospital. We refused. After all, I've had angina for over twenty-five years and there's nothing wrong with me. Finally I felt as though I could protect my first born with my strength. So he gave her some nitro, made her sign a waiver saying she wouldn't sue him if she died, and off we went.

When we got home, Pamela collapsed on the bed to take a nap—another first. At last, we are all together and the holidays were great. Pamela left a day later. I sent her off saying, "Don't worry, after a few days in California you'll be fine. Check it out when you get there and let us know." But on the flight back to LA, Pamela experienced that burning sensation again, and it puzzled me. At least I knew that she would follow up.

The phone rang as I was setting the table for the highest of holy holidays, the Day of Atonement. I picked up, and there was Pamela's voice saying she would need open-heart surgery in two days. "No, it's impossible," I said. "I can't believe it. We'll be there tonight. How can we be there tonight? Okay, then, tomorrow night. Of course we'll be there. Darling, you are going to be fine. Mommy says don't worry."

The next picture in my head is of my daughter being wheeled through the hospital halls, about to be cut open. I clutched a feather boa I brought to wrap her in afterwards, knowing how she would laugh. I never believed I could lose her. The severity was still unfathomable. Triple bypass? My husband and I couldn't register the information even as we sat through the six hours it took to complete the surgery. How could I have protected my daughter from this disease, which I gave to her? I wondered. She got it simply because we share the same blood.

I never realized the toll that heart disease would take on Pamela—physically emotionally, and spiritually. The damage it did to her beliefs and her body was extensive. She was violated, scarred and sick—everything she never could have imagined for herself. And she didn't even know the half of it yet. Over the next few weeks I watched her be the trouper I have always known her to be, but she was putting on a show for her father and me, and we knew it. We had to leave to allow her time to heal.

Eventually, Pamela started to look for cures, for reasons, for other women with heart disease, and these she found. She let everything else slip away as she immersed herself in her heart and her healing… And now here comes another book, one with valid warning, one with soulful admissions, one with truth for all women.

Thank you God for giving Pamela a mind that has helped heal her body and soul. Writing this book lifted her spirits back into the land of possibilities. Knowing my daughter as I do, I am not surprised to see that she has landed safely and healthfully into her new life. She continues to dazzle. She will inspire all those that she is able to with her *joie d'vivre*, and she will keep on going.

HEALING THE HEART

Prevention of Heart Disease in Women

By JANE FARHI, M.D., cardiologist at Mount Sinai Medical Center

More women (6.9 million) than men (6.7 million) have heart disease. So why on *Desperate Housewives*—the nation's most watched television show, a show that's for and about women—was the character that died of a heart attack a man? Was it a throwback to 1950s thinking, when all the studies and health initiatives were directed at men? Or do the writers of *Desperate Housewives* think that they know their demographics, which reveal (according to the Framingham Health Study and the Chicago Heart Detection Program) that women under forty-five rarely die of heart attacks?

Either way, I worry that the writers of the show fell prey to a common misconception among Americans today: that women need not worry about coronary artery disease; that heart disease has always been and continues to be a men's disease. This is not the case. Sixty-five is the new forty-five, and by the age of sixty-five more women than men have heart attacks. Not only is coronary artery disease the leading killer of women, but twenty-five percent die suddenly, without warning or any prior symptoms of heart disease. One-third of all heart attacks are silent.

How do we approach a disease that can be both silent and deadly? The Framingham Heart Study followed thousands of people for forty-four years, and their children for twenty years. The researchers developed a risk-factor score that has been used to divide asymptomatic, non-diabetic individuals with no overt signs of heart disease into three risk categories: low, intermediate, and high. Doctors can use this data to estimate your risk of having a coronary event in the next ten years. The risk factors that the Framingham investigators found most significant were age, high blood pressure, total cholesterol, HDL cholesterol, and smoking. For example, a fifty-nine-year-old woman whose cholesterol is 240 with an HDL—that's the good cholesterol—of forty-eight, smokes, and has blood pressure of 140 over 80 will find that she has a fourteen percent risk of having a heart attack or dying from cardiovascular disease in the next ten years.

It's important to note that the Framingham study did not investigate the following important risk factors: diabetes (because doctors assume you

have coronary disease if you have diabetes); early
family history; obesity; sedentary lifestyle; history
of drug use, particularly cocaine; or stress. It also
did not include novel risk factors such as the use of
Vioxx or hormone replacement therapy.

If you are at high risk —that is, greater than
twenty percent risk of a heart attack in the next ten
years—you should consult your doctor about aggressive risk-factor reduction. This includes, number one, taking aspirin daily. You may have read on
the front page of the *New York Times* that an aspirin
a day is *not* recommended for women. That's true
for younger women, but here's the fine print. The
Nurses' Health Initiative found that an aspirin a day
for women over fifty actually did reduce coronary
events by over twenty percent. And the average age
of the women in the study was fifty-four. Remember, women get heart disease a decade later than
men, so if the average age of women had been sixty-
five instead of fifty-four, we could expect to see even
greater benefits, probably closer to a fifty percent
reduction in heart attacks, as with men.

The second intervention concerns lowering your
cholesterol levels. This has been shown to be just as
effective for women as men. You should know your
cholesterol levels. An ideal cholesterol profile would
be an LDL under one hundred and an HDL above

fifty. LDL is the bad cholesterol, and HDL is the good cholesterol. You can lower your cholesterol levels with medications, and also by controlling your diet. Most importantly, concentrate on eating foods low in cholesterol and saturated fat and high in fiber. Maintaining a healthy weight (waist measurement of no more than thirty-five inches) and exercising regularly (at least thirty minutes, most days of the week) will also help naturally lower cholesterol levels.

Third, lower your blood pressure. Though 140 over 90 is still considered the upper limits of normal, an ideal blood pressure is below 120 over 80. In fact, recent studies show that we should be talking about pre-hypertension, which has increased risks similar to hypertension, when your blood pressure is between 120 and 140 systolic. You can lower your blood pressure with medications, and also by consuming a diet low in salt and rich in fresh fruits and vegetables. People with high blood pressure also should not consume much alcohol (no more than two drinks per day). As with reducing cholesterol levels, you can lower blood pressure by managing your weight and exercising regularly.

If you are in the intermediate risk group, meaning your Framingham score lies between 10 and 20 percent, then you should have a screening test to help define your risk better. These include cardiac

C-reactive protein, which is a measure of inflammation; homocysteine and other markers of coagulation; and ultrafast CT scans that measure calcium in the coronary arteries and can actually show plaque. A calcium score of over 80 points to significant coronary disease.

If you're in the low-risk group, you're probably like the women on *Desperate Housewives*. Except for the stress in their everyday lives, they are models of heart-healthy living. They're thin, they jog, they drink in moderation, and they're always chomping on celery sticks. As long as they don't have any other risk factors (such as genetics), they may have years of heartache from men, but the probability is they won't have a heart attack—at least not until they're much older.

But regardless of your risk category, both men and women need to pay attention to this silent and deadly killer in our midst. If only Bree had taken her husband's chest pain seriously and gotten him to the hospital sooner, he probably would have survived for another season.

HEART ON FOOD

My Cure Anything Chicken Soup

For years and years, chicken soup has seen me through all my ills. From colds to the flu, bitter winters, deep depressions, and, of course, heart trouble. I believe chicken soup is the best companion for any illness, a cure all remedy that has already withstood the test of time. It's low in guilt and rich in nutrients from vegetables (and love), it's filling and nurturing for both heart and soul.

Most chicken soup recipes are pretty similar. But I've been subtly perfecting mine for decades, adding and subtracting flavors. My chicken soup is a little of a lot of things: people who have shared their soups, my heritage, roaming the world for flavors, and a good old fashion gut response to healing. And now I firmly believe that I now have the recipe for The Best Chicken Soup on Earth.

A few tsp. of extra virgin olive oil
2 leeks or 1 medium-sized onion
2 large organic carrots
2 large ribs of celery
1 tbsp. thyme
2 8-ounce cans or boxes of

A handful of parsley, chopped
2 tbsp. coarse salt (sea salt works best)
2 sprinkles black pepper
1 whole chicken (or 2 chicken breasts). Organic is best—the taste and quality will reflect in your soup and in your body.

chicken broth   *A bunch of fresh dill, chopped*
(again, think organic)   *½ cup white basmati rice*
2 quarts water   *(optional)*

1. Take a soup pot and line the bottom with a few squirts of olive oil. Slice leeks, carrots and celery into little disc shapes. Throw them into heated oil with gusto and sauté for 6 to 8 minutes. Add thyme, salt and pepper.

2. Rinse the chicken and put the whole shebang in the pot, then create a blessing for all these ingredients before they are cooked. Sauté for two to three minutes. Add broth and about 1 to 1 ½ quarts of water, determining for yourself how thin or thick you'd like your soup to be. Praise the chopped parsley, dill, and rice as they enter the pot. You can add other flavors such as slices of ginger in the winter, cayenne pepper if you like it spicy, or whole grain noodles instead of rice. Be the master of your own soup.

3. Put on some music. Cook for two hours over medium heat, stirring occasionally and acknowledging the good job the soup is doing (soups love to get compliments while brewing).

4. Remove chicken, de-bone and strip of fat, then throw the well-tended pieces of chicken back into the soup. Serve with a crusty, whole-grain baguette (good for dunking), a small salad, and a well deserved glass of cabernet.

> ♡ *Food should always be prepared with an open heart, with love as the major seasoning.*

Heart Song

Elizabeth F., *Irvington, New York*

When I was thirty-nine years old, I started to feel poorly. I'd get tired much more easily, anxious, and sometimes short of breath. It turns out these are all classic symptoms of heart disease, but I had no idea whatsoever that what I was experiencing was related to my heart. First of all, the symptoms came on very gradually. This disease is insidious. Secondly, I did not fit the profile at all. I was young, active, and a very healthy eater. I was never a smoker or a drinker. And I'd practiced yoga and meditation for years. What I did have were five year-old twins and a teaching job at a university in New York City. So I figured my body was just responding to being under too much stress.

The problem was that the symptoms didn't get any better even when I did the right things to relieve stress. I adjusted my schedule so that I worked fewer hours and had to commute into the city less often; I went to bed earlier—nothing changed. In fact, I got worse. I started having what I thought were anxiety attacks, heart pounding and sweat dripping. And I'd get these crazy dizzy spells. When I started having trouble walking up the stairs—which I'd had no trouble climbing up and down when I was pregnant with my twins—my husband insisted that I see a doctor.

My general practitioner listened to my story and agreed that I was probably suffering from stress, but he wanted to run some tests anyway. They were inconclusive. So he said, "Let's just wait and see. Pay attention to how you're feeling." I thought maybe I should exercise more, so I started running and doing more yoga. I only got dizzier, more lethargic and breathless. Sometimes I had to grab hold of the countertop just to stand up.

Eventually, I went back to the doctor, and he sent me to a cardiologist. The cardiologist's tests were also inconclusive. Plus I didn't have any stabbing or radiating pains, none of the classic stuff. So we still didn't suspect heat disease.

Three months later, my heart was packing up and getting ready to leave. We'd been playing our game of hide and seek for long enough. The heart symptoms kicked in full force. I started having palpitations and irregular heartbeats. My cardiologist was now convinced that something was wrong with my heart, though he couldn't figure out what or why. The tests still weren't revealing anything.

Now I really applaud this doctor, because he did not let his ego stand in the way. Eventually he admitted that he couldn't figure it out, and he referred me to a pediatric cardiologist. I was thinking, "A children's heart doctor? You've got to be kidding me!" But my doctor explained, "First of all, he's brilliant. Second, he is very familiar with unusual, atypical heart conditions and defects because he delivers newborn babies who come into the world with bizarre conditions. Your heart problem could be a congenital defect. Please just go. It's worth a shot."

So I went to see this pediatric specialist in a sort of tongue and cheek manner, thinking of it as a joke. But I tell you, the moment I met this man, I recognized what an incredible human being he was. He spoke to me about my condition, looked over my files, did a few simple X-rays and CT scans, and within thirty minutes delivered my diagnosis. "I got it!" he exclaimed. "Your heart is failing and you need open heart surgery."

"What are you talking about?" I replied. I literally could not believe my ears. "I've been coming in for over a year! I've had all these tests! I'm a total health nut!"

He said, "Look lady, you're dying. Your valve is leaking terribly. Your heart is working too hard. If you don't fix this soon, you will die."

I was stunned. This whole time I'd thought, "This cannot be heart disease. I'm just not the classic candidate." Even now I can't believe it. I know that there's a family history there, but I tried so hard to make my life better that I really thought heart disease would skip me. I'm not living the lifestyle of my relatives. My father died of a heart attack, as did his father, but they ate whatever they wanted and didn't exercise. Not only that, but I have three older siblings who live more stressful lives than I do and eat terrible food, and yet none of them has heart disease. How could this possibly have happened to me, the healthy one?

But what could I do? I was dying. So in early January, I had my open-heart surgery. I was fortunate enough to have a doctor who's called "Golden Hands" because he's such a skilled surgeon. But I think it's more than that. He doesn't bring his ego into the operating room. He says, "This is the work of God," and he performs his surgery by following closely to his faith. The man has never lost a patient.

After the surgery, Golden Hands explained to me that I'd had a hole in my heart. Maybe it had been there since childhood, maybe I'd gotten it later on—we'll never know. Apparently children who are born with this defect rarely live past thirteen. So I felt very blessed. The doctor told me that my healthy habits had probably saved my life. That made me feel a little better about the fact that my chest had been ripped open and now scowled with angry scars like a warrior. It made me feel a little better about the fact that my kids had lost their innocence watching their mother fall so ill.

During the recovery process, I struggled a lot with depression. I felt so ashamed. But I came out the other side a more daring—and, dare I say, better—person. The experience forced me to re-evaluate my entire life, and I concluded that I wanted to make some changes. I left my marriage, which wasn't allowing me to grow into who I wanted to be. I left my university job, which felt too constricting, and got a real estate license. I took my children to visit our homeland, Nigeria. I've become involved with the American Heart Association, helping other women deal with their heart disease.

Here's what I want to say to you: You have to take giant steps, because this is the only life you have. You must be courageous.

4.

THE BOOK IS SEALED

I ached in the places where I used to play.

—LEONARD COHEN

I'm wrapped in a silver Mylar blanket. I died and have been reincarnated as a baked potato? I can barely breathe and my friend KT is standing over me. My mouth tastes like I just drank a mercury martini. What is that thing squashed down my throat? A day glow-colored plastic ribbed tube that looks like something out of a George Lucas film. It's suffocating me. Two more tubes sprout out of my stomach like an alien birthing itself. A gaggle more wind in and out of God knows where on my body. Machines around me beep on and off, flashing red neon numbers. I feel as though I am watching my share price plummet during the recession—it was a bad day for Pamela stock on the Dow Jones.

As I slowly regain consciousness, I hazily recall that I've just had open-heart surgery. I gag on the thought. Is that why my hospital bed is burning hot: My aluminum foil wrap is designed for cooking, not for lounging. I drip pools of sweat as if I were in one of my detoxes. If only that were true. I might be hermetically sealed except that I can still see and hear and smell. I want to vomit, but how? Into the tube I'm choking on? And worst of all, it seems that no one is as upset about this as I am.

The Heart Truth

Women are twice as likely to die from heart attacks as men. Men face a 5 to prevent chance of dying after a heart attack; for women, the likelihood of death is doubled.

—AHA, 2005

Nurses on both sides of me calmly, implacably touch, adjust, and monitor the situation. One comes in and puts a phone to my ear. She says it's my sister. When did I get a sister? I'm too tired to argue. I can't say hello, all I can muster is a grunt. How am I supposed to talk with a tube shoved down my throat? The nurse whispers, "It's okay, just make any sound." She says my sister really needs to know that I'm okay. Then I hear the voice on the other end of the line. My dear friend Donna Karan has convinced the nurses that she is my sister so that she can find out for herself how I'm doing. Most people know Donna Karan as a famous fashion designer. She's complimented throughout the world because of the beauty of her designs, and for the way she understands a women's movements while making them feel uplifted, sexy, and empowered. Putting all that aside, the way I know her best is as an *anam cara*, a soul friend, someone with a big heart and a an even bigger spirit. I moan on the receiver and she gets that I'm alive, sort of.

> ♡ *When you've got heart disease, love is not all you need. You also need financial security or at least great health insurance, knowledgeable and compassionate doctors, faith, and courage. But love is a great starting point. Don't underestimate how much the love and prayers of your friends and family can help you heal.*

The last 24 hours remained a blur. What I did remember was waving to my parents and friends with the back of my hand as the nurses wheeled me through the double doors, down the hallway of who knows. I remember my father's face pressed against the swinging door windows of the OR, tears rolling down his eyes. I remember asking God if to please do some good with me, put me on *Oprah*, help me make this a priority for the sake of all women. I also remember thinking, before they put me under, why didn't I have that ice cream cone I really wanted, was it going to kill me?

With that thought, I fell into the drugs and a kind of peace took over that took me into another life.

The night before the operation I had a strange dream. I was sitting on a chair in a room, when Celine Dion came in wearing a bright red dress and sat across from me. She stared at me for a few minutes and then began singing, "My Heart Will Go On," when she finished she shot me another look, got up and left the room. This was no time for subtleties, this was as clear a message as I could get.

Heart Song

ANITA F., *Milwaukee, Wisconsin*

Three months before my first heart attack, I went to my doctor and complained like crazy about how exhausted I was. I told him I felt bad all the time. He took one look at me and said, "Anita, you're fat, you're fifty, and you're working too much. What do you expect?" So I went home and cried and felt horrible about myself, but that was that.

Time passed… Now it was December, and I was on my way to a holiday party. I got down to the car, and I start feeling like I couldn't breathe. I was coughing to clear my throat, desperately trying to get more air. This was coming out of nowhere. So I got frightened, and since I had my cell phone with me, I called 911.

A short time later, the fire department showed up. Four strapping young firefighters come walking over and took my blood pressure, which was really high. I felt so sick. My pulse is 140. They looked at me sitting there, barely able to breathe, feeling worse than I've ever felt in all my life, and told me that because I didn't have any chest pain, I was fine. I have the flu. Then they told me that it would cost three hundred dollars for them to take me two blocks to the hospital, so I should just go home and relax. They said, "This isn't life threatening." I said, "That's okay, I have insurance. I want to go to the hospital." But they kept talking me out of getting treatment. So eventually I said, "Go away."

I thought about going to bed, but something kept nagging at me. I just knew that I had to get to the hospital. So I very slowly made my way to my car and drove the two blocks there. The parking lot for the ER was full, so I parked about a block away. And very slowly, two steps at a time, huffing and puffing every step, I started to make my way to the entrance. When I get to the circular driveway for the ER, two nurses who (ironically) were outside smoking saw me and realized what bad shape I'm in. So they lifted me past the check-in desk and start yelling for a doctor.

Once I was in the ER, they ran a bunch of tests. These revealed that I had pneumonia and was suffering from a heart attack. I was frightened. I was thinking, How could this be? I'm too young. Well, there was no arguing with what was happening. It was surreal, especially after the whole incident with the firefighters. They'd left me feeling ridiculous, like I was being a baby wanting to go to the hospital. Were they ever wrong!

I didn't call anyone that night. I think I needed time to adjust to what I'd been told. I'd had a heart attack in my early fifties, and it had been a bad one. I had pneumonia. And I needed open-heart surgery. I was just so stunned. Later, when I did tell my parents, they were not amused. I remember trying to explain that I hadn't wanted to scare them. I felt like somebody had pulled the rug out from under me and I couldn't catch myself. I felt like I was falling and falling…

I was in the ICU for a week because they couldn't do the heart surgery until my pneumonia had cleared up. There was every chance that I would not even make it to the surgery. A priest even gave me my last rites. But I did make it. And I made it through the surgery. That's life-altering stuff.

Today, I feel better and happier than I have in years. It's really, really true. I never thought that I would be grateful to have had a heart attack. But my life was not going the way it should've been going. I was working too much, I was exhausted, and I didn't feel good. I wasn't enjoying myself at all. I have turned that around enough so that now life has its rough moments, but there are lots of wonderful things that I enjoy and look forward to. For instance, I'm just so excited to get up in the morning and work out. If you'd told me two years ago that I was going to be addicted to exercise, I would've told you you're nuts! But now if I don't go, I feel like I'm missing something.

Also, I took a class in rehab called "Freeze Frame." It's a mini-meditation session. What they've found is that feeling sincere gratitude can actually make your heart rate slow and your blood pressure go down. So I learned this technique where you focus on your heart, like you're breathing through your heart, and think of something that you're truly grateful for. And I do feel grateful. I have wonderful family and friends. I've had some of the best doctors anyone could hope for. I'm very lucky, truly blessed. So I do these mini-meditations for two minutes at my desk, five times a day. It's amazing how well it works. I have the same job, but I handle it so differently. Even my arch-nemesis can't get to me anymore. I have a different attitude. People are amazed at how I laugh at things that used to make me tear my hair out. Instead of getting upset if something I do doesn't work out, I tell myself, "Okay, I made a mistake. I'll learn from it and move on." You can't beat yourself up all the time. I've always been really tough on myself. I'm grateful that I don't have that reaction any more.

Since my open-heart surgery, I've learned to take the time to enjoy things. There are mornings where I live, very close to Lake Michigan, when the sun is coming up and the sky turns these amazing colors. And I'm just so excited to be able to see these things.

The hours pass, both non-existent and agonizingly present at the same time, just like my body. I am pure pain. Everything hurts, especially my chest. Finally—minutes, hours, days later?—a doctor appears. He yanks the tubes out of my stomach, and I wince. He then pulls the tube from down my throat. That is a huge relief, like breaking a long awaited silence or screaming like a mother giving birth. I try to speak, but feel as though my voice has been taken away (I don't find out how true that is until months later).

The surgeon describes what transpired. He says they sawed me open with a real saw, and because I was so small (everything is relative, I guess), they broke two of my ribs in the process. Then a clamp pried me open like a newly formed clamshell so they could bypass my arteries. How is it possible that this is the most performed operation in any hospital? It's barbaric! He goes on to say they made a long, snake-like slice up my right leg, from my ankle to above my knee, so they could remove a vein and make it into the two arteries that I needed for the triple bypass. My veins were thin, as most women's are, but they used them anyway. Later on I would find out that because of this, blood can't flow as freely when I exercise or am under stress. But what else were they going to do, buy some veins on eBay?

He informs me that he made my chest scar a little lower than usual because he heard that Donna Karan was a friend of mine, and he wanted me to be able to comfortably wear her v-neck sweaters again without feeling self-conscious. He actually thought about this? I didn't know doctors consulted with designers on the size of the zippers they put in. Sometimes the truth is hysterical, but this time it was surreal.

The surgeon also described how my heart was held hostage for several hours on the heart and lung machine, the traditional way station during open heart surgery. An image I still can't forget. My precious little heart, sitting there, out of time and space, left alone on the Island of Devices that Modern Medicine built. My heart's task was to try and hold on, then re-enter without any complications. The surgeon tells me that the second he put mine back it took. Bam! I was breathing on my own without a hitch, heart and body reunited like estranged lovers. He says he held my heart in his hands; I tell him not many men can say that.

♡ *During open-heart surgery, your doctor will literally hold your heart in his or her hand. Find someone whom you trust, whom you connect with, beforehand if possible.*

Experts say that when the heart is removed from the body it really is like experiencing death. The separation from your heart is what many doctors believe instigates the depression that typically follows open-heart surgery. I know I believe it. Depression came into my life shortly after all this. It seems that the removal of the heart from the body also causes short and long-term memory loss, a common side effect of this operation. I wished for months that I could have lost the memory of this event, but no, what I forgot were names of movies, people, and other seemingly important things. I could not download information that I knew I knew, which felt terribly frustrating and confusing. Maybe my brain had decided I no longer needed that stuff. Instead of instant messaging it was instant deleting. Maybe my subconscious already knew that it was time to make room for new wisdom, new habits, and new insights. Anyway, what choice did I have but to spin it that way?

The days in the hospital blended together, from nausea to morphine drips, from changing catheters to the changing of bandages, the changing of nurses, to the ever present changing of moods. Different hands, different meds, different pains, different meals, none of them good. Everyday, answering all sorts of questions with yes, no, a little, and everyday asking when and always why why why?

♡ *You're on the right path if you don't know what's going to happen next. That's called a God shot! Have faith.*

My parents were there for all of this. They cried when they were not around me; I could see it in their eyes. They took to behaving like the CNN news scroll. Every fifteen minutes, they would walk into the room and tell me how wonderfully I was doing and how successful the operation had turned out. My chest and my heart disagreed. I felt like I'd just given birth, except there was no baby for us to celebrate. Whenever friends came to visit, trying to cheer me up, I saw the look of horror on their faces. They couldn't be blamed. My bandages oozed, my chest scar bubbled up pus and other strange bodily secretions. The palette of olives, yellows, and reds that covered my body and reflected the grey-green pallor of the hospital lights hardly matched my fashion sensibilities. My friends, like all people, were drawn to the gore, looking at me with a combination of love, horror, and disbelief. But I have to say my parents really pulled it off. Thank God for the acting gene that is so dominant in our family. We played along with each other just like we always had. They never left my side except when my friends wanted an audience with me alone. Everyone wanted to hold my hand.

♡ *Hand-holding is the closest we can get to heart-holding.*

Heart Song

SHARAMI K., *New York, New York*

The medical profession failed her. Yes she was obese but that is not a reason for bad care. She had chest pain and shortness of breath which they called asthma. She had been complaining of chest pain for two weeks. She said that her EKG was normal, but she was sent to the hospital in an ambulance, kept overnight for cardiac enzyme tests, and sent home with the same symptoms. Again, she went back to her doctor. Now they told her that it was her gallbladder so she called me to discuss gallbladder issues when they sent her home with an antacid medication.

My sister knew that we had a history of heart disease in the family including me, who had had a heart attack and heart surgery five years earlier at age fifty-three. If she were a man, she would have had an angiogram in almost any hospital in America. There is a practice called standard of care that the medical profession should follow in all situations, especially when medical insurance is not an issue. Any nurse that I asked said that they couldn't understand why they never did an angiogram. But, nurses have also seen the prejudice expressed in private about obese patients. So they look for problems relating to food and blame the symptoms on diseases relating to food.

The day before Thanksgiving she had a stomach procedure that required anesthesia. We spoke that night and she said "I'm so tired that I don't think I can make it to my bathroom." I spoke lovingly and said "Annie, stay home and rest tomorrow. Your friends won't mind if you don't go to Thanksgiving dinner." Two hours later, she was dead.

Her sons insisted on an autopsy and I agreed. We all needed to know what happened. When I found out, I was devastated. The LAD, left anterior descending artery had closed resulting in sudden death. My LAD had also closed, but I lived and she didn't. It became a spiritual question that I am still answering. I believe that when it's time, it's time. But on the other hand, with proper medical care, does that change anything?

At the house after the funeral, her neighbor said he wouldn't go for medical treatment in Las Vegas if his life depended on it. He went to Los Angeles for medical care. I wish that she had known it. I wish that my sister had listened to me about women and heart disease. I'm glad that a friend of mine did listen, did read the book *Dear Heart* and did save her own life by calling 911 with a sudden onset of chest pain.

To you, dear reader, please, listen to your body; respect what you need, in fact, demand that you be treated properly by learning what you can about women and heart disease. You may save your own life as my friend did. I'm sorry that my sister couldn't.

Three times a day, I shuffled down the Maalox Hall of Fame saying hello to my fellow heart-mates. No one but me was under seventy, so each day (given what happens to the memories of heart patients seventy and older), I heard the same thing over and over again, "What is a young woman like you doing here for an operation like this?" This seemed to be the most-asked question about me, replacing the previous FAQ, "So when are you going to get married?"

The doctors seemed to feel the same way. I was the favorite viewing specimen for the many med students studying cardiovascular disease because I was the best headline their teachers could have ever wished for: Healthy Woman Taken Down in her Prime by Heart Disease! That drew crowds.

I had a fabulous male nurse, Aaron, whom I adored. He kept me company every night when I couldn't sleep. Sleeping in a hospital is impossible; there is no such thing as sleep or humility when you are a patient. There is fear, there is projection, there is second-guessing, there is denial, and there is rage, but there is no rest for the rest of you. What's more, the meds kept me in a constant state of nausea. So in would come my knight in shining armor to amuse and distract me with a copy of the *Enquirer*. He'd read me the idle celebrity gossip, share hospital stories, and never ever forget to tell me how well my healing was progressing. It's a real gift that nurses have; they know how to make you feel better no matter what else is going on.

My progress was measured in two ways now: bowel movements and breathing. In order to be released, I had to prove that I had mastered both without the assistance of nurses or machines. After years of perfecting these very same skills alone, it was a novelty to have to try so hard—and then to be graded for my performance. One night Aaron showed up after being summoned by the floor nurse at four in the morning for my first bowel movement, something I can honestly say I haven't needed a witness or assistant for since I was three. It felt like I was passing a kidney stone, or rather a toxic torpedo, yet Aaron was thrilled beyond belief. This was my turning point, he said. Where was I turning towards from a bowel movement? The pain of eliminating all those meds and fears and toxins in one big movement proved to be greater than that of having a zipper sewed into my chest. I was sweating and crying and exhausted, partly due to the pain but also to celebrate my freedom, my imminent release into my new "normal" life. What a dump it was.

The Heart Truth

Forty-six percent of female, versus twenty-two percent of male, heart attack survivors become disabled from heart failure within six years.

—WOMENHEART. 2005

Then there was the breathing. Three times a day we played a game in which I had to breathe into a tube containing a ball. Having practiced yoga and meditation for decades, I felt I had perfected the breathing thing. But breathing with broken ribs and a slice down your chest is kind of like doing yoga with a watermelon tied to your back. The object of the game was to get the ball up the tube, thereby clearing my lungs of the idle debris that had filled them during the trauma. I was determined to win this one every day, as if there were a free car or trip to Maui as a prize.

What I did win was an upgrade to the Liz Taylor suite. After the ICU, this was a palace, complete with dining room, kitchen, and Liz's own assortment of take-out menus from taco to pizza places. Food was the last thing on my mind. Nausea was always first, while walking and moving came second. Night after night, I sipped ginger ale as if it were a vintage bottle of cabernet while sucking and picking the salt off my saltines in an attempt to conquer the unyielding sensation of seasickness. I was lost at sea, miles away from my usual carrot juice and tofu.

May I take a few moments to vent about how bad hospital hygiene products are? The way they feel and smell is beyond my comprehension. Take note: Everything that is antibacterial and antifungal, is also antisocial. Sometimes they give you a product that tries to smell like mangoes or coconuts, but the actual odor is lethal for patients with nausea, like me and most others recovering from surgery. For the $150,000 it costs for the operation, you'd think they could throw in a gift basket with a few Aveda products!

I had a window off to the side of my bed that I stared out

of for hours each day, marveling at how people were moving around, getting in and out of their cars, carrying flowers to the loved ones they were visiting—and doing everyday tasks with such ease. How had I turned into the visited one? How had I become the one immobilized while others got to run around? How did this little portal become my world?

It was on one of my many sleepless nights that I finally got up the courage to look at myself. Like a novice stripper, I peeled my robe off shoulder by shoulder and let it drop to the floor in front of the full-length bathroom mirror. I figured Liz must have done this a thousand times so I was in good company. It was there in my reflection that the new Pamela came into view, the one with all the markings that made her look as if she'd been initiated into some long-lost island tribe, my cashmere skin branded like a new calf.

The Heart Truth

After menopause, women begin to develop and die of heart disease at a rate equal to that of men.

—AHA, 2005

I was trapped day after day in waves of incredible sadness but still could never manage to cry. Not once since the day they told me I had to live by different rules. Not when I was alone at night, not in between visitors, not after they said I would be on medication forever, not even when I caught the first glimpse of my new and very forever scars. Not even one tear.

I tried to think about my future but never got far. I was at the end of the vision that I'd always had for myself. You would think that I would have felt overwhelming gratitude after having survived an ordeal such as this, but to me life was now a burden. Who asked for twenty more years like this? Who would want it? Who was I to refuse it?

When a woman undergoes heart surgery, she must come to terms with her longing and the way it will be doused. Heart surgery has a particular flavor to it that is never really discussed— the flavor of bittersweet chocolate. You get a bitter truth and a sweet revelation about your life. Caution: a little goes a long way. Naturally I did not know then what I know now. But I came to see that all my bravado, ego, and past performances meant nothing to the inner workings of my heart. My fears ruled while my faith faded. In the end, my courage was really just leftover endurance.

♡ *You get a glimpse of a person's true character when all is lost, when the bag of tricks no longer prop up the play.*

After two weeks in the hospital, the doctors let me leave. My mother and father came to live with me. I was in their custody yet again, only a little more battered and bruised than the newborn they had carried home forty-seven years earlier. I had to take a regimen of medicines to slow my blood down, and the beta-blockers turned me into a slug. I drank soups and teas up the kazoo, morning, afternoon and night. My friend Miriam, the tea master, blended a bunch of amazing blends to soothe me, and they did. But each morning I took a survey by looking around the room, and each day the same question popped out: "What am I supposed to do now?"

There was nowhere to go and nothing to do. I'd never had a moment like that before in my life, and now suddenly I had thousands of them strewn together. Since music has always been my indoor version of nature and has defined so many of the important moments in my life, I felt that I needed to listen to love songs, especially torchy ones. Sound tracks are as important to look forward to as they are to look back on. I listened 24/7 to the same mixes, absorbing love and pain into my heart. It was as if it were the first time I could feel this intensely. Could it be true that my clogged arteries had blocked off my feelings as well as my blood? Could it be that this blockage had led me to make choices in my life that I could now change? Music became my words, my emotions, the way I defined time. Music was my background to stare at the life that had fled somewhere between the saw and the scar.

♡ *Time goes slower when you are healing, so you must fol-low. Speeding allows you to overlook those parts of you that have been hiding for years.*

My dear friend Geneen came to care for me. She tended to

me better than any nurse ever could have. She was there from the beginning of this saga until the end because that's just the way she is, and thank Goddess for that. She became the clearing station through which everything and everyone from the other world had to pass. KT, my parents, various visiting nurses, and even Dr. Jesse took part in the revolving care and love I received. Some days that was comforting, and some days it became claustrophobic. I felt more like a caged cougar than a princess being waited upon hand and foot.

Friends and business acquaintances called constantly and sent flowers and cards every day, but even as the gifts and tokens for healing multiplied, I struggled to find my voice. It kept getting lower and deeper. Eventually I asked Geneen to leave a message on my answering machine saying, "Thanks for calling. While I very much appreciate your thoughts and concerns about me, I cannot return your call at this time." I felt like I needed some freedom and some time to myself. Two weeks later, my parents had to leave. I needed to grieve, and grieving in front of one's parents is not an easy thing to do if you are the one who traditionally enlivened. I could not keep up the charade of getting better when inside I felt like I was dying.

KT sent over a masseuse who sings as she massages. She thought the combination of music and touch would help me revive. That sounded as normal to me as it probably sounds crazy to most of you. Remember, LA has a reputation to keep up. She began to sing me a lullaby as she laid me gently on the table like a newborn. She touched me in soft strokes and sang her heart songs angelically, stroking my scar over and over, until there she found it, the oil well of tears, and opened the floodgates to my sorrow.

I started to sob in waves, like the ones breaking outside my window. I sobbed for past, present, and future pains. I sobbed as though I were mourning someone close to me who had died, and had begun to realize that someone was me. I sobbed like I was in the presence of something sacred. I sobbed like I had never let myself sob before. The masseuse read my scars as if they were Braille. My body responded to her touch as if I was an instrument and music was the language we could both understand. This kind and unusual stranger brought me home to myself with a love song, probably one that had been playing inside me all along.

♡ *Music a wonderful medicine for the heart: It involves romance, memory, dreams, and movement—all of which are stalled for a while in recovery.*

HEALING THE HEART

My Top Ten Healthy Heart List

Oz Garcia, Ph.D., Celebrity Nutritionist and Executive Chairman, OZ Wellness Corp.

The way I approach heart health is through nutrition. After seeing thousands of women in my practice, I recommend adopting the life-lengthening strategies that have served the people of Crete and Okinawa so well for generations. In fact, a 2007 study found that both men and women who consumed a Mediterranean diet lowered their risk of death from both heart disease and cancer.

Here are my top ten recommendations for maintaining a healthy heart:

1. Eat a liberal amount of fruits and vegetables
2. Eat generous amounts of fish or shellfish at least twice a week
3. Consume healthy fats such as olive oil and canola oil
4. Use herbs and spices instead of salt to flavor foods
5. Eat small portions of nuts
6. Drink red wine, in moderation
7. Consume very little red meat
8. Exercise for at least twenty minutes every day
9. Restrict your calorie intake one day a week
10. Take a fish oil supplement

HEART ON

It Was Always You: A Poem

So I am searching for my deeper voice, the one inside me that rises for my screams and shrinks from my whimpers. The voice that's sure of what she knows. The one that drowns out the voice that is frightened and clueless on this new journey. I need this voice now; I need her to help me live the everyday. I should be able to draw on her like water from a well. Instead, I am drowning.

With pen in hand I, am dominated by her voice, my muse who has been with me for so long. Typically we meet only for as long as it takes to put the words on the page; then we part like lovers after the affair, running back to our normal lives, our regular partners. Never speaking a word about the time together.

The wordsmith in me always waited impatiently for her visits.

But things have changed since the surgery. I no longer have patience. Our relationship has become tempestuous. There is no room for meandering about the dark holes inside searching for her. I want her to be available to me—on demand and on target. I fear that impersonators have already taken control. They hold her hostage, trying to keep my neuroses agile.

I first met my voice at age twelve when a yearning for poetry overtook my body like a religious fervor and carried me into a frenzy of words, pouring images onto pages, staining me with myths and romantic illusions.

I have not been as generous with her as I have with my daughter voice or my ego declarations or my lover's whisper or my big boss bellow. They have been my favored children, the voices that got me the scholarship, the money, the success, the voices that prospered the more I orphaned her. But what was I to do? She wanted to make a poet out of an entrepreneur! It never would have worked. Nevertheless, we continued to meet time and again, always passionately, always briefly, over the next forty years.

Now that I have been to death's door, I have that different sight. I want to say it as I see it. I want to be more languid with her, this strong partner inside me. I'd like to travel for a while through her deep voice, cavernous with echoes. I want to know who she is. Is she sexy? Earthy? Eccentric? Does she bathe or shower? Does she cook or order in? Does she judge or accept her fate? And is she at peace with popping in and out of my existence? She has been calling on me for years, and yet just when she caught my attention, she hides herself away.

Where are you, deep voice? The diminutive giant goddess that undulates from my tongue onto the page, that makes me strong, that gives me faith. I am looking for you, and won't rest now until I find you.

Heart Song

CHRISTINE G., *Central Islip, New York*

My story is quite common with the exception of one thing: My age. I was just twenty-seven when all this happened.

It was March 16, 2005, a Wednesday. I'll never forget that day for the rest of my life. I was at work doing my normal routine, but I wasn't feeling too well. I'd been to my regular doctor the day before because I was coughing a little and had been experiencing some minor chest pains. She'd said I probably had an upper respiratory infection, and so had put me on antibiotics. Usually, these gave me major stomach cramps, so that day I waited until an hour before I was going to get off work to take them. But only twenty minutes after taking the antibiotics, I already had terrible cramps! My boss told me to go ahead and leave.

At that exact moment, I started to sweat profusely, to the point that I had to take one of my shirts off. I felt like I needed to get fresh air because I couldn't catch my breath. So I grabbed my jacket, pocket-book, and keys, and started walking briskly down the hall. As soon as I got outside, I collapsed. I fell to my knees trying desperately to catch one single breath but I couldn't. I was so scared. I thought I was having some kind of crazy reaction to the antibiotics. Just then one of my co-workers passed by and saw what kind of condition I was in. He ran to call me an ambulance. (Thank God he wouldn't let me leave! I lived only five minutes from work and would've tried to drive myself home.)

The first official on the scene was a police officer. He gave me oxygen and told me over and over again that I was having an anxiety attack and I needed to calm down. At this point I was not only sweating and couldn't breathe, but I also had stabbing chest and back pain that would come and go every couple of minutes. I started to think I was dying. I told my colleagues to call my husband (who was working about two hours driving time away) and my sister-in-law.

When the ambulance finally arrived, the EMTs said the same thing about having an anxiety attack. Now I had no idea what anxiety felt like. I'd never been in the hospital before and nothing serious had ever happened to me. But I knew this wasn't psychological. I just knew that something wasn't right! So the ambulance driver took me to a hospital about fifteen minutes away, where my sister-in-law was waiting for me. As soon as they took me out of the ambulance, I told her I thought I was dying. My chest hurt so bad that I still couldn't breathe.

In the ER, the doctors and nurses hooked me up to all sort of machines and did a bunch of blood tests. They couldn't figure out what was going on. They wanted to know if I took drugs and I said, no! None! I kept telling them that I was having massive chest and back pains, and I was obviously experiencing shortness of breath and sweating like crazy. I told them that heart disease runs in my family (my father had triple bypass at forty-seven, my uncle had a heart attack last May). They even hooked me up to the EKG machine about six times within four hours and my results were completely abnormal. And yet still they didn't diagnose me with a major heart attack! They were simply in denial because I was so young.

When my parents and husband finally made it to the hospital and saw the poor shape I was in and that the staff was doing nothing for me, they got really upset. My father told them to give me an aspirin because it sounded like I was having heart problems. Finally the cardiologist came in. As soon as he hooked me up to the EKG he figured out what was going on and gave me aspirin and rushed me to a cardiac hospital. It turns out I'd been having a massive heart attack for the past five hours! The staff at the cardiac hospital was waiting for me when I arrived, and they sped me immediately to the OR to have a stent put in. I later found out that my arteries had been ninety-five percent blocked.

I've only just begun my journey down the long path to recovery. It's been nine weeks now since the surgery. I feel very frightened but at least I'm alive. I've been doing online research to find out about my disease, and that makes me feel better. And I've gotten a ton of support from other women with heart disease in chat rooms online (see appendix for more information).

I now know that the doctors and nurses in the other hospital had no knowledge about heart conditions in younger people. I had every single symptom of heart disease in women. They just did not want to believe that I was having a heart attack because

I was young, athletic, ate well, didn't do drugs, and weighed only 130 pounds wet. But I'm here to tell you that if it can happen to me, it can happen to anyone. So believe your body when it doesn't feel right. Don't let the doctors try to talk you out of it. *You* know best.

5.

THE THREE STOOGES
OF HEALING:
Disbelief, Denial, and Depression

When you give up hope, your heart goes as well.
The heart is the most poetic organ in the body.

—DR. MEHMET OZ

I was tired, very, very tired. Exhaustion permeated my whole being—exhaustion from what had just transpired, exhaustion from what had been my life so far. I never slept anymore because I couldn't turn right, left, or onto my belly. I'd never mastered sleeping on my back and my open chest certainly didn't make it comfortable to move any other way. I was riddled with pain that radiated throughout my body. Days and nights were a blur. My body felt like pizza dough without the toppings, flattened and pummeled.

I had a cavernous and excruciatingly painful hole in the middle of my chest snaked with the outline of a scar. The ribs that had been broken during surgery didn't appear to be in any hurry to mend, and my usually high spirits had lifted themselves up up and away, leaving no note to indicate their return. I felt like a Jack-in-the-box, the kind you play with when you're three years old. Pop goes the weasel! The weasel, it turned out, was depression.

The Heart Truth

**Depression and the heart are sisters.
Depression is a common warning sign of a heart attack,
as well as a common consequence of one.**

—Dr. Galina Mindlin

Depression is an insidious and indiscriminate visitor. It doesn't knock, pick a good time to drop by, or wait for an invitation to enter. It doesn't dress in bright colors or crack jokes or have an expiration date. It simply shows up and nestles in like a long awaited guest, lounging on the sofa. Depression has no single personality trait. It camouflages itself within its host. So you don't know until you have it whether it'll make you eat or sleep too little or too much, cry all the time, or get angry. The only constant is the changing moods. It can feel like a goose-down blanket, but it also can feel like a gossamer nightgown that clings to the skin for dear life. Depression can be handled but never thrown off entirely. It permeates a life like a carbon monoxide fume, deadly and invisible to the eye but always apparent to the heart.

♡ *Depression is measured by its weight not height, and it's usually heavier than the person carrying it.*

Heart Song

Sharami K., *New York, New York*

When I was fifty-one years old, I experienced real depression for the first time in my life. By that I don't mean I felt sad for a few days or so. It was as though a gray veil was hanging in front of my eyes. I tried to shake the feeling, but realized when I didn't want to water the plants anymore that something was really wrong. As a therapist, I knew that I needed help. I started taking an antidepressant for a few months. This treatment helped me change a difficult situation for the better, which changed my need for the meds. So I stopped taking them.

A couple of years after this depressive episode, when I was fifty-three, I began having dizzy spells some mornings. I also noticed a lot of indigestion. I used over-the-counter drugs for heartburn to combat the indigestion. I ate a bigger breakfast for the dizziness, which I thought was related to the hypoglycemia (low blood sugar) I'd suffered from in my youth. When I started to experience shortness of breath going up subway steps or hilly streets, I attributed this to being out of shape. In retrospect, if any of my friends or clients had described these symptoms to me, I would have immediately suggested that she see a physician. But in my own case, I viewed each of the symptoms individually rather than collectively. So often, we don't listen to or help ourselves in the careful, attentive way we would another.

About six months after these feelings began I had a large heart attack. It was a Saturday morning in October of 2000. I was in my kitchen talking with a friend when I got dizzy and almost fell to the floor. My friend helped me sit down and drink a glass of orange juice. About 20 minutes later, I felt better. We had breakfast, my friend left, and I went about my day.

That Friday I went to see my primary care physician for a previously scheduled visit. I mentioned the dizzy spells and indigestion in passing. She did an EKG and shocked me when she said, "My God, you've had a major heart attack." The heart attack had occurred when the largest coronary artery, the left anterior descending (LAD), had closed. I was told that 75 percent of people who have that artery close die instantly. I felt how very lucky I was and that clearly, in my language, "it wasn't time." I had more work to do here on this planet.

My physician wanted to know why I hadn't come to see her sooner. I can only answer that it's a woman's issue. Most women don't pay attention to the signals their bodies are sending, but would pay attention if any of their family members had similar symptoms. Perhaps it is part of the Superwoman complex that women have of being able to scale tall buildings and get through everything for everyone in a day.

My new cardiologist ran a battery of cardiac tests, which revealed that I needed bypass surgery. Since only one artery had closed, we were able to wait several months for the surgery. During that waiting time, my cardiologist kept asking me if I was depressed, saying that depression is common after a heart attack. I would always say no. But then one day I noticed that gray cloud returning and recognized that I was becoming depressed again. Only this time the depression felt deeper; it felt like it was in my body, not just my mind. I began to take Celexa daily, which had the remarkable effect of getting rid of the depression rather quickly. I felt emotionally better but still physically very tired. I stayed on Celexa until the day before the heart surgery, and then discontinued it to see if I would need it post-surgery.

Actually, after the surgery I felt ecstatically happy to be alive. I said a prayer of gratitude each morning when I awoke and each night before I went to sleep. I valued every day more than I ever had before. My life was fine as I healed from the surgery, and I went back to work. But then four months after the surgery, there was the depression, back again. It was clear that it was not situational, as my life was wonderful. It was brought about by my heart disease. I went on an antidepressant again and continued to use it for almost two years. I also feel that it took almost two years for me to fully recover from the heart attack and subsequent surgery. When I felt totally like myself again, I decreased and then discontinued my use of the antidepressant. While I no longer take the medication, I am grateful for having had it in my time of need.

Today my heart is functioning well and so is my

life. In fact, a month ago I was so happy that someone told me an overabundance of joy could hurt my
heart. I told him, "Please include that in my eulogy
some day."

Mine was a virgin depression. Never having a bout of it before, I found it seduced its way into me, making me feel oddly
reassured at first. It started with me idly staring out my window
for days, not able to be or do much else. I took this to be serenity
at first until it fixed itself into not being able to do much else. I
stared at the ocean and the sky until I was blind—blinded to my
past, blinded to my dreams, blinded to my new reality, blinded
by the sun. I was most assuredly blind-sided by the pain, both
internal and external. I stared outside so much because I did
not want to have to look at what was going on inside me. And
yet the more silent I became, the more animated my depression
grew. I became sensitive, cranky, teary, bitchy, grouchy, sad, and
pessimistic: the seven dwarves rolled into one. Worse yet, I soon
discovered that I had no control over it and, no ability to stop it.

They say all you need is a crack to let the light in; Leonard
Cohen has a song about that. Well, I had a cavernous and excruciatingly painful hole in the middle of my chest big enough for
a lighthouse beacon, yet still the darkness was victorious.

My depression gave me an entirely new personality. It was low, quiet, and very negative (*quell surprise*)—all opposites of the old me, what I still thought of as "the real me." This persona had no identity yet. She didn't cook, sleep, shop, or laugh. I didn't even know the simplest things about her, such as what she liked to eat or wear, or how she got things done. But somehow she had *become* me. Me, the über foodie, the one who used to stock her refrigerator as if it were wartime, now had lost her appetite for everything. Me, who had loved life so much, now seemed able to think only of death. Nothing fit anymore—my clothes were too big, my voice was too low, my body was a mess. I felt as though I was trapped in a carnival Fun House, but certainly without any of the fun.

The Heart Truth

Individuals who suffer from depression are four times more likely to have a heart attack than those who aren't depressed.

—National Institute of Mental Health (NIMH), 2001

My illusions about health, happiness, and love lay scattered in a million pieces like a broken plate on the kitchen floor. My only hope was one day these beautiful bits of mosaic would come together to create an artistic form for my new life. Each day, though, became another foray into a place that had more and more doors but fewer and fewer exits, more questions but never any answers. I would lie in bed every night—still and opened like a new bride—wanting to be captured. I was waiting for an image, a voice, or a message to tell me what my next steps should be. But nothing and no one came. I started thinking about death all the time—not like committing suicide, but rather in the sense that dying felt like the logical next step. That thought surprised me and left me feeling very agitated.

♡ *Having heart disease is like giving birth or falling in love:*
   You have to be ready for whatever it brings.

I honestly had no desire to do anything but sip tea, stare at the ocean, and watch *Oprah*. Thank heavens for Oprah; she can lift anyone's spirits. She is definitely Everywoman's soul mate. Her make-overs delighted me, her investigations into what's was really going on engaged me, and the pureness of watching people emerge with a transformed spirit, inspired me. Unfortunately, *Oprah* occupied only one hour out of twenty-four in a day. Why can't we have her replace the non-stop news on CNN?

Where was a good news and network when I needed one?

Weeks after returning home from the hospital, I felt that I could not tote the wheel barrel of my depression any longer; I was a 100-pound mule with a 500-pound load. I had no references for the way I felt, no one to confer with about it, no fashion forecasters to tell me what to wear for it, no other women in my age group to call up and cry with over it, no support groups that I knew of with whom I could share my story. Here I was, my heart split wide open, and there were no takers. I felt more alone than ever.

> ♡ *When you feel your path is bleak or that your soul has made a mistake, hold on a little longer. Your real journey is stretching out its course. Time is a stranger where healing is concerned. But in the end, your heart will find its way home.*

I had to go in for post-surgery checkups weekly. All the machines and all the doctors were happy with my progress. We seemed worlds apart in our thinking. The fourth week I went in, when my depression had fully taken over, I had a moment of grace. After the testing was complete, my nurse, Susan, closed the door.

"Pamela, how are you doing really?" she asked. "I mean *really?*" She said "really" as though it were a code word for us to speak honestly.

I replied, "Susan, I am depressed all the time and I can't shake it."

She nodded her head. "Yes, I know, that's what happens."

"What do you mean 'that's what happens?'" I asked.

"To people who have had open-heart surgery," she replied.

"Why is something like this being kept secret? The doctors told me I'd be on the golf course in six weeks. It's already been four weeks and I don't remotely know how or want to play golf!"

Susan smiled and came closer. Softly, she asked if I wanted some meds to help me through this difficult time. She must have done this a thousand times before, and yet she said it in a hushed tone of voice, as if a drug transaction were taking place. "What kind of meds?" I asked, intrigued.

"Antidepressants," she said. "You would only have to take them for a while, just until you feel back to yourself."

"What if I never feel back to myself?" Recently, I'd come to accept this as fact.

"You will, don't worry," Susan said soothingly.

"How would I know who my 'self' was anymore, even if she did come back? And if I take these meds, how do I know these meds would not take me further away from myself?"

Susan put her hand on my shoulder. "Please think about it," she urged. "You don't have to suffer like this."

"Don't you feel that ship has sailed?" I replied.

Susan then suggested an anti-anxiety drug or some pills to help me sleep. I refused again. I honestly did not want anything to help take the edge off—been there, done that. I said I would give it another two weeks and then reconsider.

Why, after years of popping pills, wouldn't I agree to take some now on the chance of escaping this horrible depression? The answers were:

a) I did not believe in them.

b) They scared me.

c) I liked the depression.

d) All of the above.

Heart Song

RACHEL G., *Boston, Massachusetts*

Ten years ago, when I was forty-six years old, I started feeling fatigued. I'd worked out for twenty years, wasn't overweight, didn't have a cholesterol problem, ate decent foods, had never smoked, and so most of the risk factors for heart disease weren't there. I did experience some discomfort in my forearms from time to time when I was walking up a hill or doing an aerobics class. But I never had any chest pain, so I didn't make the connection to my heart.

This went on for several weeks. Then one day I had to turn around during a walk and come home because the pain in my arms got so bad. I lay down on the couch thinking it would get better, but instead I began to feel worse. Then out of the blue a picture popped into my head—I really believe in the grace of God, let me tell you. I saw this diagram from a medical book I'd read years and year earlier, a drawing of a man that showed where you might have pain during a coronary event. And I remembered that it showed pain coming down the inner arm. So I thought, "Could I possibly be having a heart attack?"

I went to see my doctor, and he sent me to a cardiologist who did a stress test. He saw some irregularities on the EKG, but wasn't sure if there was anything wrong. So he had me do a local cath at the nearest hospital. When I was done, he came into my room and said, "You need a bypass. You have ninety-five percent blockage. But just a single artery." I was a workaholic, running my own business, always go, go, go. I said, "I can't have a bypass. I have seminars to lead this week!" But my husband, who was in the room with me at the time, looked at me and wept. He had just lost both his parents and his brother at age fifty-three, so he was scared to death. I was not scared at all. I'd had a number of abdominal surgeries for endometriosis, so I was cool and collected.

For my surgery, I went to Mass General, the leading hospital in the area for this type of work. I had to wait three days for the bypass. It went well, and I only had to stay in the hospital for five days. Then I was anxious to get back to work. I wanted to show everyone that I could bounce back, do everything that I had done before. I wanted to prove that coronary heart disease had nothing to do with me. I wanted people to say, "Isn't Rachel a whiz?"

Recovery was very frustrating because I had to exercise so slowly and methodically. I wanted to run faster, work out harder. I thought, "This is ridiculous." But I was my own worst enemy. While I did well taking it easy for the first eight weeks or so, after that I was off to the races. The problem was that I was never okay with the idea of having heart disease. I thought, "That's for old people, people who are fat, people who don't work out, and that's not me." Psychologically, I was not very accepting of myself. I wasn't giving myself what you need after you've gone through something like this.

So I went straight back to working round the clock, exercising hard, drinking too much. I wanted so much to be carefree, to do what I wanted. And almost a year to the day later, I wound up in a psychiatric facility. I was clinically depressed. Not only was I ignoring my heart experience, but also I was having issues with my mother's psychiatric health and grappling with my own long road of infertility that had come to an end with a hysterectomy. I was grieving, working like a lunatic, and taking care of both my parents. It was too much responsibility. Any normal person would have said, "No, enough is enough." But it's that woman's side of me, the people pleaser, always wanting to take care of others but not myself. So I wound up spending five days in a lock down psych hospital. And I needed to be there.

After that, I did a pretty comprehensive stress management program. In the past, if there was something I didn't want to think about, I'd always dive deeper into work and that would make me feel competent. Through the stress management program, I learned the value and techniques of meditation. That helped a great deal in my recovery. I believe that meditation can be the answer for someone as stressed out as I was. Because if you get to that place where meditation takes you, then you're living mindfully, so you'll be more likely to exercise, eat well, set your priorities, and take care of yourself. I still struggle with stress and workaholic tendencies, but if I stop and meditate twenty minutes a day it really helps. I also started taking antidepressants, which were a great relief.

It's been ten years now since my heart surgery, and there have been a lot of ups and downs. I'll make slow progress, then slip again, then make more progress. I'm still struggling with my need to prove myself through work, be entertaining and smart. But I have a new attitude. "What's the point?" I ask myself.

I've sung in the church choir ever since. Music really grounds me; it helps me feel more in touch with myself and that which is greater than I am. I don't drink anymore. I'm tired of cooking so I still struggle with eating well, but my weight is normal because I watch my carb intake. I work out with weights now as well as doing cardio. I do yoga. I take cholesterol-lowering drugs. I do everything that I should do to stave off another cardiac event.

I'd love to tell you, "I've arrived." But I haven't. In my own mind I'm still always trying to prove, trying to prove. I tried even harder after the bypass and it landed me in a psychiatric facility. And yet at least I've managed to simplify my life. I sold my dad's business. I'm trying to think about working less, maybe dropping to twenty-five hours a week. On one level, I want to have more space and air in my day, but on the other hand I'm fighting a constant battle with myself because I'm such an urgency addict. "Ooh, I need to go here, I need to go there," I tell myself. Many women do that. I definitely do.

I need constant reminders otherwise I gravitate towards things for which I'll be reaffirmed and acknowledged. I want people saying, "Isn't she smart? Isn't she great?" It's that ongoing need to please everyone and make everyone think you're so cool. It's a sickness actually. I know from experience, from my depression and psychotherapy.

It's life or death. I could wind up back there with a heart attack. It could happen. I still have the same genes, and I'm still under a lot of stress. When I hear myself speak like I'm speaking to you now, then it reminds me that I have to change. I have to slow down. But it's a lifelong process, getting your head screwed on straight when it comes to taking care of yourself.

Let me say right here and now that no matter what specific type of heart surgery you have, you will never be the same—not necessarily better or worse, more conscious or less sympathetic, thinner or heavier, there is really no judgment about who inside you wants to emerge in the end. Part of you *will* emerge, though, whether or not you like her, want her, or think you need her.

I'll say it again: No matter what, *you will never be the same*. Why can't they (the doctors, the nurses, the websites, the healers, the ones who've been through this before) just tell you that?

It's a disservice to the soul of a person not to communicate the alienation she will feel once her heart is tampered with. What are they so afraid of, anyway? I mean it could be very exciting to think, "After this surgery, I am going to be different. Great! I needed to be different." What a boost, what a bonus to the trauma: The promise of seeing changes in your self. A new self, one who won't bore you, ridicule you, harass you, or even diminish you. One who is up for a change and takes on the challenge willingly. Why not? Why can't they tell you *that* before they dim the lights?

Well, I'm here to tell you that something really does happen to you once your body is cut open. Whether it's molecular, physiological, or emotional, there *is* a significant change that occurs, and it *is* real. Do not let anyone tell you otherwise. You are the one who experiences the differences inside yourself. As women, we react in body and emotion. I mean when was the last time you heard a man freaking out over his thighs being too heavy? We are different creatures, and—most of the time—neither male nor female doctors can morph themselves into our body experiences. Please, honor what you feel. Trust yourself. People who have met you for the limited number of hours it takes to have an operation don't know you or even have the time to know you. Certainly they can't know you the way you know yourself.

♡ *Instinct is that essence of thought untouched by our*

*schemes. When you have heart disease, it's more important
than ever to listen to your instinct.*

Since I didn't want to take meds—not that there's anything
wrong with antidepressants, they just weren't what I was pulled
towards at this point in my healing process—I turned to Dr.
Jesse. She proposed a number of ways for me to try to relieve
these overwhelmingly dark feelings: herbs, breathing exercises,
positive imaging. They ran the gamut of alternative thinking.
And they did help, but they did not cure.

So I forced myself to look a little deeper. "What makes you
really happy, Pamela?" I asked myself. "When no one is looking,
what truly satisfies you?"

It was with that question that all my voices suddenly reappeared and orchestrated a climatic moment. There it was, the
kernel that popped, the idea that got a rise out of me just like an
unexpected kiss. The question is always better than the answer.
Sitting on my rocker waiting for *Oprah* to make my day, having
a bowl of chicken soup, Sage at my feet, wearing my cashmere
sweats, that's when it entered. I heard it distinctly, enunciated
perfectly: "DO NOTHING. DO NOTHING, PAMELA."

Never before had I connected with *wanting* to do nothing or
thinking that was an answer to anything. I had always wanted to
do *more*. More was my significant other. It was now the spring
of 1999 and DO NOTHING was going to be my personal way
to ring in the new millennium. I had to allow that to be the

most intuitive part in answering my call, for I had nothing else to go on.

> ♡ *Be content to be and not do, especially while you're heal-ing. Remember the lessons of kindergarten: play for a while, and then nap and have a cookie.*

Two pieces out of those hundreds on the floor suddenly began to make sense and come together. In fact, they were a perfect fit. I could stare, write, sip tea, walk Sage, paint, cook, watch movies, sleep, and eventually *heal*. Oh my God! What a concept. I could slowly come into a new rhythm that would not only serve my health, myself, my life, but also allow my depres-sion its due. I think this is what most people refer to as balance. I did not opt for the antidepressants; I opted for the "Do Noth-ing" prescription. This was the medicine I could stomach, and so I wrote the script.

We heart women need to get rid of the stigma surround-ing depression. We really do take everything to heart. That is our birthright as women, and we must live it and sometimes act it out. Why should we be made to feel that there is some-thing wrong with us if we suffer a bout of the blues, especially following such a traumatic event? Why do we think that we have to run away from our depression, mask it, or rename it? Taking medications are definitely the ticket for some, but for others it can prevent you from venturing in and enjoying the ride. Why is it that we think that sadness is the part to fix in ourselves, while happiness is our true destination? Why do we try to *think* away what we *feel*, when inside we know it has never ever worked that way? I think the Beatles said it best: "Let it be, let it be." Whichever method you choose to assist you, make sure it's yours: Your decision, your wish, your nature. It's *your* healing process, after all. It's *your* heart.

The Heart Truth

Depression may make it harder for you to take your meds and follow through on other treatments for heart disease. It can also cause chronic elevation in stress hormone levels, further damaging your heart. Don't be afraid to diagnose yourself and seek treatment for your depression.

—NIMH, 2001

HEART ON

An Excerpt from My Recovery Journal

It is almost three weeks since the operation and the vagueness around the reality still surrounds me. I still wake up at 5:15 thinking "blood pressure, temperature check." I still feel shocked by the baby steps I take to get to the bathroom, when I once walked with such stride. I still feel that horrible nausea in my stomach as if I swallowed more than I could chew. I still feel like crying my eyes out every time I like at the line down my chest. The mark of so many bypasses that are taking place at the same time.

Days pass by long and empty, but what is different about healing time is that it belongs to nothing else. It is not beholding to schedules, ambition, or compulsion. You must give up all notion of the life you are leading to surrender to the life leading you. How phenomenal a discovery at forty-seven.

The depression comes each day to teach me the value of the nascent internal movements that have no place to go. I get to be out at sea and just trust the course. The tears are not the cleansing ones yet. They are tears of a former life and loves, of times gone by. But I do feel a clean sweep of sorts beginning, as if cleaning up and putting in these new arteries will not allow any of the sludge from the past to resurface. I feel like somewhat of a recluse in my feelings, yet a strange comfort in the company of them.

HEALING THE HEART

Music, Emotions, and the Heart

By GALINA MINDLIN M.D., PH.D. in Neurophysiology and Neuropsychology, Assistant Clinical Professor of Psychiatry at Columbia University

Depression, anxiety, and stress all contribute to heart disease. Negative emotional states create a domino effect inside the body: cortisol levels skyrocket, your arteries constrict, your immune system slows down, your heart rate increases, your blood pressure climbs. Over time, these unhealthy responses take their toll in the form of disease (especially heart disease and cancer) because your body simply cannot bear the stress. The tighter you hold onto your emotions, the more damage you do to your heart. Learning to control your emotions is therefore one of the most crucial keys to a healthy heart. You've got to be able to let go, give up the fight, and take a break.

It is especially important for women with heart disease to mediate their emotional reactions because their hearts are so vulnerable. Yet as women, we generally rely on our feelings to negotiate our way through life, so this can prove quite a challenging task. Furthermore, women with heart disease tend to be Type A, meaning they need to be in control. Yet when they have a heart event, they lose all control. Their response to this lack of control triggers stress, which causes more symptoms to appear and eventually exacerbates the disease itself.

Whenever there is turmoil or chaos in your life, make an effort to be calm, act calm, and bring calm into your body. Before confronting a known stressor such as a bad boss or a bad marriage, first try to get yourself into the zone—one in which you feel calm, centered, and ready to take on whatever life brings your way. You can accomplish this through meditation, deep breathing, exercising, getting some sunshine and fresh air, reading poetry, giving someone a hug, singing, laughing, or spending time with a pet, among many other options. These activities immediately help counterbalance the effects of stress by relieving tension, quieting the mind, slowing your heart rate, reducing constriction in your blood vessels, and lowering levels of stress hormones.

While many doctors and psychologists overlook this simple method, I highly recommend listening to music. Music frees the mind and reduces pain. Thousands of years ago, the Greeks and Romans used music as therapy. Today, music has been found helpful in treating heart-related ailments such as high blood pressure, unstable angina, and depression, and in speeding recovery from surgery. Clinical trials demonstrate that women and men who listen to music during operations have a much more positive outlook going into surgery and experience of the situation.

There is no stigma associated with listening to music, it has no negative side effects, and nowadays it is highly portable. So why not give it a try? Once you see the benefits of music in terms of relaxation, you realize it is an ally both in preventing disease and in reducing symptoms inherent to any diseases you might already have.

Keep in tune with the mind and the heart will follow. The mind is the bandleader and the heart is the orchestra; it's really your choice how and what you play.

HEART ON
A Poem and A Prayer

In this pit
I am reaching out
My fingers seem blurred
And tired
I am tired
Of crying to myself
I miss you
You who lived as me
With my name and spirit
I want you back
I need you near
But I don't know your name
I've changed addresses since we last met

I now live in a place called need
Need?
a crowded place
So lonely,
so full of itself?

These labored thoughts
Trick me into
*   receiving your call*
The one that invites me into
*   continuing*
Through
*   this paradox*
Of doing
*   And doing without*

Heart Song

BETH M., *nurse practitioner and holistic healer,*
Sag harbor, New York

I've owned a holistic women's health care practice
for the past twenty-two years. I do a lot of work

with hypothyroidism, adrenal fatigue, and heart disease. And I've wondered for a while, what's going on with women and their hearts? My professional opinion is that our modern lifestyle places too much strain and stress on us. We don't take enough care of our health, in the holistic sense of mind, body, and spirit.

But what I want to talk about specifically here is a very common problem among women known as Broken Heart Syndrome. A study published in the February 2005 *New England Journal of Medicine* confirmed what I've known for a long time to be true: a tragic or shocking event can produce classic heart attack-like symptoms such as chest pain, shortness of breath, rapid heartbeat, and fluid in the lungs. Fortunately, recovery from Broken Heart Syndrome is physically much easier than recovery from a real heart attack. But the emotional recovery is an entirely different story. And I have a story of my own about BHS that I'd like to share.

About four years ago, a wonderful man came into my life—or so I thought. I was fifty-seven years old at the time. He decided that I was his true love and announced that he wanted to spend the rest of his life with me. He was married, but he left his marriage when I said I wouldn't see him unless he was single. We had amazing times together sailing and skiing and sharing life emotionally and physically. Things started to get serious and we were making plans to spend our lives together. I had finally connected to my soul mate, and the future looked very fulfilling. It seemed a miracle that at this point in my life I was going to have some real happiness.

Then it all fell to pieces. One day I asked if he was seeing anyone besides me. He said he was— many other women, I was soon to discover. Not only that, he confessed that he was going to strip joints and getting lap dances on a regular basis. This was very upsetting to me because I'd waited a long time to be with someone, and I honestly believed he was the love of my life. I didn't understand how he could do these things.

When he first told me about the other women, I started crying hysterically. I felt betrayed and unsafe. My heart rate rapidly escalated to 173 beats per minute. I went to the cardiologist to have a stress test, and he told me that I had ventricular tachycardia. He said that if I didn't go on meds immediately I could go into heart failure. I was terrified. The next morning, I went to the drugstore to get my beta-blockers. But I didn't want to take them. I was seeing an expert homeopath and a naturopath at the time, and so I decided this was the type of treatment I preferred. I didn't buy the drugs; I got myself a stuffed panda instead. When I got home, I called my natural medicine practitioners and was given a homeopathic remedy to calm the heart. I also took some natural hormones to balance the hormones that had gone haywire from the stress response.

After conducting extensive research on my own, I found out that the stress response is a major contributor to heart disease. Yet most practitioners seem to focus on diet, exercise, and laboratory numbers without discussing the stress hormones and their effect on the heart at all. I realized that I had Broken Heart Syndrome. You see, when you're under stress, your body puts out huge amounts of cortisol and epinephrine. These stress hormones make your heart beat rapidly and create a hormonal imbalance. I knew that the only way to cure myself was to end the relationship. So that's what I did. My "true love" admitted that he was a sex addict and was not willing to seek treatment, so

I suggested he go back to his wife who could pretend not to know. And that's what he did.

To me, this story is such a vivid demonstration of the mind-body connection. Look at what an addictive relationship, devastation, and depression can do to your heart! Staying healthy and preventing heart disease is not just about getting proper nutrition and exercise; it's also about managing your stress. This is the whole basis of my practice with women. I'm working with what I myself must learn. But my experience, as awful as it was, has helped me encourage my clients to take a good look at their lives and their relationships. Avoiding illness is not just about taking meds; it's about changing your life. If you don't, you *will* get sick. I had to let go of this relationship in order to save myself. My lover wasn't willing to give up his addiction, and I wasn't willing to give up my heart.

Let me make a cautionary statement here. One of the reasons why women get misdiagnosed when they are suffering from heart attacks is because doctors tell them that they're just having an anxiety attack. If you're having symptoms of heart disease, please don't just dismiss them as due to Broken Heart Syndrome and stay home. Go to your doctor and get tested. It's entirely possible that you do have heart disease and need professional care. At the same time, I think that when people have heart attacks, doctors should ask, "What's going on in your life, in your relationships?" Because stress hormones are so powerful, they really can change the dynamics. I've seen it with cancer, too. They suppress your immune system. There's always a bigger picture.

My heart problems haven't come back at all since I got over that man. I'm dancing, I'm having a good time, I feel healthy, I look younger, and I feel younger. So remember: I'm not saying you shouldn't have your heart checked out just because you're going through some life trauma—you always should. But keep in mind the critical link that exists between your heart and everything else that's going on in your life. Each exerts a powerful influence over the other.

I'm not down on love these days. Love can break your heart, but it can also heal your heart. Now that I've had this experience with Broken Heart Syndrome, I'm able to help other women heal better. I'm able to look at their physical as well as emotional symptoms with deeper compassion and insight. And in the end, the goal is always healing.

6.

THE WHITE SALE: EVERYTHING MUST GO

If you are irritated by every rub, how will you be polished?

—RUMI

Slowly, like clouds burn off on the June gloom mornings in Malibu, my depressive fog was beginning to see light. Either that or it was becoming an integrated part of the emerging new me. I felt a deep longing to return to some semblance of my old, familiar life. The problem was that as soon as I began to recover from the physical and psychological hardships this trauma had put me through, I was knocked flat on my face by financial hardship. It is often said you are one illness away from losing it all, and here I was with my one. What can stop a person who would never stop before? Take away her health and then her money at the same time. The one two punch that will render you helpless. I'd been distracting myself, allowing denial to set in, but high noon had arrived in red ink. Quite simply, I was broke.

The Heart Truth

**Bypass surgeries can cost more than $150,000,
not including all the extras.**

Where had all my savings gone? I was three years and change into the healing process. There were so many exceptional expenses: medicines, vitamins, and herbs to counter the horrible side effects of the medicines, numerous alternative treatments for body and spirit, and checking in with countless doctors to get their opinions on why this had happened to me. Not to mention all the usual expenses: rent, car, food, pet care, insurances galore, and so on. And the fact that I hadn't earned a penny for some time now all landed me in trouble.

Heart Song

Mary D., *Kansas City, Kansas*

I used to be a runner. I used to teach aerobics classes at several different levels. But ever since I got heart disease last year at age sixty-three, I can't do that stuff anymore. I don't have much mobility. I cry a lot. And I've completely run out of money.

My heart disease showed up out of the blue. I was in the middle of an advanced aqua aerobics class when my heart rate shot up to 170 and would not drop. The doctors diagnosed me with arterial fibrillation and performed two surgeries. I wish I knew what caused it, but I don't. No one has a clue. The cardiologist wants to implant a pacemaker now, but I won't allow it. I feel like it would mean killing a large portion of my heart.

I have really struggled with the lack of a support system. Many of the important men in my life can't or won't deal with my heart disease, which has resulted in my having more emotional and psychological problems. You've got to look for a female support network. (See the appendix which offers resources for women with heart disease.)

I've also had a terrible time dealing with health insurance. People with chronic issues frequently can't get health insurance. Or if they did have it, they are dropped. The only thing that saves them is if they can get on a group policy under someone else's name. I have tried some of the "low-cost clinics." But I find that these doctors just want to get you out the door as quickly as possible, so they tend to over-prescribe medications. Now the best doctor who will see me is 63 miles away, and the closest ER that will take me without health insurance is forty minutes away. I guess that's just the way it is.

It's true, money can't buy you health (or love), but it *can* buy what you need to survive and live on, especially health care in today's world. And I had an entirely different definition of health care than most people. I had an exquisite yoga teacher, Micheline, who studied how heart patients should move after their surgery and helped me reconnect with my body in a respectful and empowering way. I did Pilates and weight training to strengthen my muscles, cardio by walking on the beach with Sage, and chi Qigong to maintain my inner balance. I had hands-on energy work and acupuncture, and for that extra assurance all the new modalities LA had to offer. I had colonics to purify me and Indian hot oil massages to soothe, I had my skin rolled, a process whereby the masseuse basically pinches every part of your skin and pulls it away from the bone to keep it vital and supple. My friend John, an extraordinary aromatherapist, the Shaman of Scent as I call him, concocted scented oils to help diminish my scars and keep my spirits alive. I worked with a dream interpreter to decipher where my internal process was taking me. I did it all until it put me back together again.

♡ *Since as women we all come with the same parts but different operating instructions, disease and recovery work differently for each one of us.*

Diet-wise, I naturally shopped the cornucopia of organic foods at the farmer's market every week. My food staples consisted of fruits and veggies, soups, and whole grains as always, but I had started desiring more protein—fish, chicken, and even a lamb chop or two. I'd been a healthy eater for decades, but now I gave myself a wider berth to explore. Never a chocolate fan before (yes, I know that eliminates me from the Women's Club), I became an avid connoisseur of dark pure bittersweet chocolate. I even introduced soy lattes after being a tea drinker for so long. And after years and years of not drinking, I also started to enjoy a glass of red wine here and there, as the doctors recommended for my type of heart disease. Slowly, these helped me regain my appetite for life.

The Heart Truth

**Wine (no more than two glasses per night) and dark choco-
late (at least 70% pure) are pleasant dietary recommendations for most women with heart disease. They both seem
to help with blood pressure and cholesterol. Enjoy!**

——DR. JESSE HANLEY

The standard meds that doctors prescribe for post-surgery
heart disease patients were not for me; I had some kind of reaction whenever I took them. There is no such thing as a standard
regimen for women with heart disease anyway, just as there is no
such thing as a standard hormone treatment that works for every woman. There is a protocol that doctors usually follow, but
not everyone fits into those guidelines. I was, as usual, a misfit.
There has still not been an all female research project on meds,
incredible in 2009 that we are still looking at 200 lb males as
our norm. That said, I convinced the doctors to let me try red
yeast rice, a more natural version of Lipitor, to help reduce my
cholesterol. My cholesterol went down sixty points.

In addition, I did chelation treatments. The substance EDTA
is injected into your blood via an IV drip for two-plus hours
each session. It then binds with heavy metals (such as lead) and
the plaque they leave behind, thereby helping your body secrete
these unhealthy elements through your urine. Although there's
no FDA approval for chelation and the sessions left me shaky

at times, I still believe in it because it worked: my angina symptoms began to diminish.

So, yes, all these treatments cost money, sometimes lots of money, and insurance doesn't cover most of the alternative approaches. The realities were pressing in; I had to get back to work. If only I knew what I felt like doing, or was capable of doing, then I could proceed forward. But I had no clue.

Now that death had come knocking and I had no children, I felt more certain than ever that I needed to leave a legacy behind. I wondered what my gifts and passions could conjure up before I left this planet. I'd always believed the greatest gift I had was the way I could inspire people to change. I'd lived my life in non-stop change mode and now, looking back, knew it to be my greatest teacher. I also believed that women are the most amazing catalyst for change. I've had the pleasure many times of creating events where women could gather to listen and share their stories. Storytelling is one of the oldest healing tools in our culture, throughout time it has been the way women gathered information and gave advice. Because in every woman there is a story and you know she wants to tell it. The story lives in her heart, and the story never ends.

I wondered if I might find a way to make this a reality: to bring women together in order to effectuate change. I imagined that my new way of looking at life might bring a perspective to all types of women.

Serendipitously, I connected with my old friend Carole, a successful film and TV producer. We had known each other for over twenty years. She shared my vision, and had been doing her own workshops with women, mothers, daughters, teens all the sizes and shapes we come in. She was exploring the relationships we all assumed and how we played them out. What a perfect fit, so together we began developing a plan to bring both our ideas to fruition. Carole knew me in the years when my magic was still available, so working with her was not a reminder of what had just happened but rather a confirmation of the Pamela Who Can Do Anything. And that was the Pamela I needed again now.

♡ *The soul, if given the chance, will stay dancing with you to the right end.*

Heart Song

CAROLE ISENBERG, *Pamela's close friend,*
New York, New York

It was the summer of 1981 when I first met Pamela. I was living in Los Angeles and Pamela, who lived in New York, was visiting one of my close friends.

She was a sprite with short dark hair, luminous brown-cherry eyes, a wide, disarming, bucktoothed smile and big energy. Pamela was designing unique jewelry in those days. But she was always looking at the alchemical nature of life, seeking the opportunity to express herself in as many creative mediums as possible. We clicked right away; the way people do when you speak the same language. My mother was dying of breast cancer and there was a lot of shame attached to the disease at the time, but Pamela didn't mind talking about it.

As we lived our busy lives on separate coasts, we kept in touch. But our contact became more and more sporadic and for several years we lost touch completely. And then one day there was Pamela on the phone, her familiar husky voice telling me she was moving to LA. "I have decided to change my life," she said. "How fantastic!" I replied. She promised to call once she was settled.

Well, I didn't hear from her for six months and when she did call she had quite a story to tell. Not possible, I thought, not possible that Pamela had triple bypass surgery. We made plans for dinner. I remember pulling up to her house in Malibu. She was tan and sitting on the front step waiting for me. I got out of the car and walked over to her and we hugged a big hug. Then we pulled back and took a good look at each other. Pamela was more woman and less sprite. She was wearing a bright green v-necked t-shirt that showed off the thin line of her scar. It was her own beauty mark.

As we rekindled our friendship, I saw that Pamela's heart event had had a profound effect on her life. The Pamela I met in the eighties wanted to be everywhere and do everything. No so this woman. There was fragility to her energy now. She was careful about how much she put out and how many people were around her at a time. I found her more thoughtful, introspective, compassionate, and humble.

Having a close friend with heart disease has been an education for me. I did not realize that heart disease was the number one killer of women. I did not know that the signs of a woman having a heart attack were different then a man's. I take stress tests regularly now and I'm very aware of any new research being done. Because of Pamela, I truly understand what it means to live a heart healthy life.

Heart disease isn't a condition that is cured. You

don't just go on as you did before. Heart disease is a condition that you live with forever. It is, as Pamela says, "a new normal." But this isn't necessarily a bad thing. I feel that as a survivor, Pamela has greater appreciation for the simple fact that she is alive—and so do I.

After five years in LA, I felt like I was getting sick of the life light, the sun, the salsa, and the smoothies on a daily basis. Maybe being in LA was just too reminiscent of everything, too much cell memory here of recovering from my heart surgery. I needed to pull a geographic recovery and cleanse my palate.

♡ *Our hearts have everything to do with what our minds imagine they conceived.*

Around that time, Carole and I began working on a project together with Revlon and Almay called "Making Up," a series of vignettes we performed on how women transform themselves from the inside out, from their make-up to their emotions. It was just the kind of program that could grow into something more substantial about inner and outer beauty. We were smitten with the idea of performance art as a way to spread information.

Spending time in NYC for the demonstrations, I realized how much I missed my family and how much I missed the Pamela I was when I lived there, PPH Pamela pre-heart. I longed for real bagels, the sounds and sights of NY'ers with their constant costume changes, the cooking smells, that waft of the streets, and the command I felt in navigating it. Dorothy had it right: there's no place like home. So with that thought, I packed up LA, got a camera, and drove across country with Carole. I had dreams again in my heart and hope on my horizon.

The Heart Truth

One in two African-American and Latina women is living with heart disease.

Well, it turns out my memory of New York City was much better than the reality of what it—or I—had become. As soon as I returned, I started to question my decision. As it turns out you never really can go home again, or at least, this was certainly true for me. The grass was indeed greener on the other coast. I found myself longing for the softness of LA, the palm trees, the humidity-free sunshine, and the calming sound of my Malibu waves. I remembered how slowly I moved there, so contrary to my constant rush down the streets of Manhattan. Here, my heart quickened at the noise, the commotion, and the smells of garbage in the August heat. In spite of the pain I'd suffered there, the West Coast had provided me with healing space, room to breathe and see my life without the drive and clutter that NYC had always embodied in me. I felt like I was neither here nor there, yet again.

Being in Manhattan immediately revved me up to a pace that I knew I could not sustain. I thought that by returning home I'd be able to reconnect with the places inside myself where I was powerful, successful, and effective. But that was magical thinking—and I was no longer a magician.

I have met many women who think the way to the heart is to chart its course rationally, eat the right food, reduce stress, and exercise. While these are all important parts of the prescription for a healthy life, they are by no means the only ones. For me, if the obvious cause of my heart disease was my family history, the secret cause was the way I metabolized stress. I cooked it up as drama and gobbled it down like a gourmand devouring a loaf of hot crusty bread. Then I'd let it stew inside me for days, even weeks, like a mastered Bolognese sauce. When I stowed my stress away, guess where it landed? Smack dab in the middle of my heart. So here I was again, letting NYC do what it does best—stress me out. I feared and felt another episode coming on, as most heart patients do, and I was right.

Heart Song

LEESANN S., *Palm Desert, California*

My story is a little different. I don't have "heart disease," per se. Rather I was born with three holes in my heart. Until I had heart surgery at the age of ten, I would literally turn blue whenever I exerted myself too much. My early life unfolded under all kinds of restrictions. I wasn't allowed to run, play, or laugh like other children for fear that it would over-burden my heart. I wasn't even supposed to cry! When something bad happened that upset me, my grandmother would hold me throughout the night to make sure that I didn't break down and start sobbing. Sometimes I'd fall asleep on one shoulder and my mother would fall asleep on the other, and we'd spend the whole night that way until we had to get up for work and school. It gave me a very strong sense of family. I feel so blessed for all the sacrifices my mom and grandparents made for me.

I'd always wanted to dance. When I was four, one of the girls at our church gave me a pair of toe shoes.

I put them on, walked over to my mom, who was doing the laundry, and said, "I'm going to be a dancer when I grow up!" My mom stopped putting the clothes in the washing machine and looked at me. "That's never going to happen," she said. But I just looked right back at her and said, "Yes, I *am* going to be a dancer." She said, "You have a special heart. But we're going to try to fix it. We're going to meet some doctors and you're going to have an operation. But that can't happen until you're older."

When I reached age ten, the doctors were finally ready to perform the surgery. They didn't want to wait too long because they didn't think I'd live past twelve, but they also couldn't do it too soon because they knew it would be a real shock to my system. They were right. It was a difficult road to recovery. My lungs collapsed and I got pneumonia, so they had to redo the surgery. Then the very next day I remember the doctor saying, "We have to do tracheotomy." They had me packed in ice. It was intense.

Well, I don't know where it came from, but the will to live was so strong in me. I was ferocious. My defiance saved me. I was able to direct it in a very constructive manner towards recovering from my open-heart surgery. I kept saying to myself, "I'm going to live, and I'm going to do what I feel called to do. I'm going to live *my* way."

As soon as I was well, I discovered to my sheer delight that my problems were solved. My energy levels increased exponentially. No more restrictions! I was free to run, laugh, play and cry. And I became a dancer for life. I started taking tap lessons, baton lessons. I'd say to my girlfriends, "Let's do that dance from *Mary Poppins*!" and we would, and I'd think, "Oh my gosh, I can really do this now!" To a child who couldn't do any of this before, it was a really big deal. I even majored in dance at college.

When I was in my mid-20's, I came to a place of peace inside myself. I realized that my heart was strong. It didn't have to do with the physical strength; it was the strength of having something greater, the strength of my heart being not just me. Our hearts are connected to the planet, the planet is our mother, and the planet has a rhythm. The essence of nurturing is universal. The strength of the heart doesn't come from the one it comes from the many. Those may sound like clichés, but they're so true for me.

Now I'm 50. My lungs still aren't real strong. I

can't run fast, and I never learned to swim. But I can dance. When you're dancing, it's not just you. There's God, there's the music, and there's what you're giving back to whoever is watching. You're being carried. To this day, I consider myself a very heart-oriented person, and have dedicated myself to helping others. Interesting how a calling can be born of what's missing sometimes, isn't it?

I was told when I was ten that I'd never be able to have children. But in college I had a bunch of tests done, and they told me that I would. What a blessing it was to hear that news! My son, Evan, was born with a heart condition as well, though not as serious as mine. He has pulmonary stenosis, which means that the artery going into his left lung is slightly narrower than the one going into his right. He's going to have a stent put in, but it should all work out just fine. Thankfully modern medicine is way beyond where it was when I was little. My husband, Jacob, and I tell him that he has a very special "lion's heart," because his heartbeat is so loud that it sounds like a lion's roar!

If you'd like my advice for how to deal with your heart issues, here it is:

1. Always ask for help from the "unseen worlds" (angels, healing entities, spirit guides—whatever you like to call the denizens of that vast domain).
2. Find what you love doing, and do lots of it.
3. Find a doctor or specialist who you really trust.

7.

WHERE IT STOPS,
NOBODY KNOWS

Let life happen to you. Believe me: life is in the right, always.
—Rainer Maria Rilke

It's Thursday, December 18, 2003 and Christmas is every-where. Even with the whipping winds, shoppers swarm the city, fearlessly navigating the thick grey applesauce slush cover-ing the streets. Store windows overflowing with fancy and fat-tening foods flirt with people's pre-holiday resolutions. Colorful cashmere temptations along Madison Avenue are crying for a communion with my inner addict. Horns honk and traffic crawls, we are immune. In other words, it's business as usual in NYC.

But for me it's not business as usual as I set off to negotiate my way through the elements to meet my new cardiologist, Dr. Jane Farhi. Much as I'd like to deny it, I've been having chest pains again. So here I am, antsy waiting in a waiting room an hour and counting for my appointment, when all I really want to do is bolt , window shop, and sip on a frothy cappuccino. Some things never change.

♡ *Heart disease is forever.*

At last I get to see the doctor. Dr. Farhi is charming, smart, and attentive. I can tell within two minutes that we're a good fit. We speak about my old and new symptoms, and I am struck by something she says after reviewing my chart "You have advanced arteriosclerosis." By this she doesn't mean that I belong in a gifted or master's level class, but rather that, having had my first heart event at age forty-seven, it's likely that my heart disease will return again and again. I also take it to mean that I'm looking at twenty more years of life at best.

Next, we proceed to the treadmill for a stress test. Two minutes, five minutes, I'm still feeling all right. But at eight minutes, I start to feel distressed. Dr. Farhi suddenly gets pale and looks up from the machines. "We need to get you to the hospital immediately," she says.

"Why, its really not so bad just a little discomfort?" I reply, face flushing. This can't be happening again.

" It looks like you might be having a heart attack."

"Right now?" I counter.

"Yes, right now," she repeats, as she gets paler and I get more agitated.

"You mean right this minute right now, or it's coming? The anticipation is the hardest part."

"It's sort of like hearing a tornado approaching without being able to see it. You notice the colors change and the air takes on a claustrophobic demeanor. There are changes in the EKG," she explains.

"How does a heart attack get so close?" I ask.

She shows me the graph. There is a big blip, but there are so many blips. I start to break down. "How can we be sure? I cannot do this again, I just can't. I won't make it."

I burst out crying. Dr. Farhi tries to comfort me and her own eyes fill with tears. She says, "I have no choice, you have no choice. We both know the truth. You are in danger of a heart attack now, and I won't let you go home. You must go directly to the emergency room. This can't wait." Does she think it's the first time I've heard this line? I am no stranger to heart disease. I know the routine. What I want to know is who screwed up and put Groundhog Day in the middle of December?

What is the difference between heartache and heart disease? Answer: the emergency room. It wasn't the hospital part that I feared, but the room beyond it, the operating room. I had just about all that I could take. If a cat has nine lives, how many does the human heart have? And how much more could I take? That seems to be the million dollar question in this lifetime.

> ## The Heart Truth
>
> **Thirty-five percent of female, versus 18% of male, heart attack survivors will have another heart attack within six years.**
>
> —WOMENHEART, 2005

I ask to forgo the ambulance. I've done that before and discovered that it's not as much fun as it looks. So I walk slowly out the door, feeling so disappointed in myself, as if I had everything to do with this, and frightened that it is another ending. A heart attack for Christmas, the gift that keeps on giving. I climbed into a taxi. "Lenox Hill emergency room, please." Still independent to the end.

> ## The Heart Truth
>
> **About half the time, bypass grafts clog up within a few years, angioplasties within a few months.**
>
> —AHA, 2005

Needless to say, I survived the episode. And now on my record, it shows I did have a small heart attack. The doctors put a medicated stent inside the piece of artery that had re-clogged.

They said this stent would defy plaque build-up and stay open longer than the non-medicated type. They were wrong. It was twenty-four hours of anguish for me, yet I got to check out of the hospital the very next day. Yes, apparently the operation is as simple and routine as taking out tonsils. At least that's what they tell you. Nothing can make me believe it, no matter how fast or how well they perform the procedure. I was exhausted for weeks following.

I started to sink back into depression. Remember the heart and depression are sisters; they know when the other is in trouble. The problem was that I'd spent the last five years denying that I really had heart disease. I had written off the bypass as a fluke. It had seemed the only way to move forward in my life. But now, with this petit heart attack and stent procedure, I couldn't lie to myself any longer. The walls of my denial came tumbling down. Humpty Dumpty was in pieces again.

But a few weeks later, I discovered that underneath all the panic, pain, depression and frustration, there was a real Chanukah gift waiting for me at, of all places, the waiting room in the doctor's office. What a metaphor. During a follow-up visit with Dr. Farhi, I met a woman who told me about her *five* stent procedures. She said, "What choice do I have? I've learned how to *live with heart disease and be positive about it.*" I felt as though this was the long-awaited message that needed to be delivered to me, a message I could finally hear. A message I chose to embrace.

Hearing the words, "learned to live with heart disease" come out of the mouth of another heart patient rather than from a doctor authenticated my experience. It didn't erase my depression but added color, like a kaleidoscope, to my ever-changing emotions. Somehow I could finally accept that I was a Heart Survivor and feel okay about it. I knew that I was a strong, capable individual carrying heart disease along with eight million other women I'd never even met. I felt a surge of energy from the realization in a way I hadn't since this all began.

♡ *Allow enough room in the agony of recovery for the ecstasy of being well.*

I realized that I would have to finally learn how to deal with my own stress. I knew for sure without a shadow of a doubt that stress was my enemy. I was still an over-the-top responder to events in my life. I would have made a great fireman but as a heart patient, maintaining this instant alert system was not in my best interest. Why could I not give each event a minute to soak in before reacting to it? What did I have at stake with this behavior? And so at long last I taught myself all the things I'd taught *other* people for decades: how to center myself, how to breathe, how to let go. "Calm down," I would tell myself. "Is all this worrying worth what it's robbing from me? Do you want to give yourself another heart event?" That last thought usually stopped me in my tracks.

In addition, I discovered a fabulous support network, Womenheart. I hooked up with a group of female heart survivors, and had monthly lunches. It was love at first bite. These women were embracing, funny, informative, inclusive, and nourishing. They were the real deal and my heart felt at home.

Heart Song

FAITH T., *Orange City, Florida*

I'm forty-eight years old now, but I started having problems with my heart when I was about twenty-one. The problem was that at age sixteen I was diagnosed with hypothyroidism (meaning my thyroid wasn't active enough), and so my doctor put me on thyroid replacement medication. Then I moved from Florida to Chicago, so it was five months before I got to a doctor for a check-up. During those five months, I lost about fifty pounds, had no energy and was very sick. It hurt to swallow, it hurt to eat. The doctor discovered three goiters growing around my esophagus because my thyroid had become overactive. He gave me surgery to remove the goiters.

At the same time, I started having a lot of chest pain and heart palpitations. I went to see a cardiologist. He told me that during this period of thyroid hyperactivity (due to the same drugs that had given me the goiters), a valve in my heart had been damaged. He put me on meds; I don't remember what. I took them because I was young and stupid and didn't understand anything.

Two years later I moved back to Florida. I kept going to cardiologists because I was experiencing the sensation of someone grabbing my heart, squeezing it for thirty seconds, and then letting it go. That would happen a few times in a row. At first it was every few months, but over the years it progressed to the point where it was happening daily. I went to a bunch of different doctors, and they tried all kinds of meds, but nothing helped. All they could tell me was that my tests looked normal and they couldn't explain what was going on with my heart.

When I first went to the doctor I have now, he asked me about my family history. When he realized that my father had suffered three heart attacks by the age of sixty-five, he said genetics had probably contributed to my heart problems along with the drugs I'd been inappropriately treated with in my youth. He did a cardiac catheterization and prescribed some new meds, which has helped. It's the closest any doctor has come yet to fixing things with my heart.

Heart disease has definitely affected my life. For one thing, I get tired out extremely easily. Trying to hold down a full time job is very difficult. Just walking across the office and back I get so winded that I have to sit down for a few minutes to rest. I'm also very aware of my own mortality.

Luckily, I was able to have children, which was a great surprise. My husband and I had tried for four years to get pregnant, and then one day it just happened. It was scary because it was only five months after the goiter surgery and it was supposed to be at least a year, but he's a great kid, as is my daughter. I have a four year-old grandson now. Because of him, I'm careful to monitor what I eat, exercise, and keep the extra weight off. I want to be around to watch him grow.

HEALING THE HEART

Nutrition for Heart Disease

BY SALLY KRAVICH, holistic nutritionist, author of
Vibrant Living: Creating Radiant Health and Longevity

I've studied health and longevity modalities from
around the world: the Amazon, the Middle East,
Eastern Europe, Fiji, India, and here in the US. In
my bicoastal practice, I've worked with women for
over twenty-five years to improve and integrate the
health of body, mind, and soul. Usually I meet with
these women in person to find out their goals and
put them on a program of stress management, exercise, food, and nutrients for optimum wellbeing.
Here I'm going to present you with a few general
rules that apply to most women with heart disease.
However, please consult a physician before implementing any major lifestyle changes.

- *Food*: The food that you eat must have the ability
  to be broken down, absorbed, and eliminated by
  your body. Here are a few rules to live by, which
  I call non-negotiable:

1. Get rid of all man-made products. Avoid all fake
   sugars, fake sweeteners, fake creamers, fake ice

cream, and margarine. These products don't have the enzymes contained in real foods, they are insoluble fats, and so our bodies can't break them down. As a result, they tend to form cysts and clump up, contributing to illnesses like heart disease, tumors, and cancer.

2. Eat plenty of fresh fruits and vegetables. I recommend consuming at least six to eight servings of veggies and two to three servings of fruit per day. Veggies are the repairers. They build new cells and provide nutrients to ensure healing. Fruits are cleansers. One word of caution: People on heart disease medications (eg, Coumadin, which is a blood thinner) sometimes are told not to consume a lot of dark, leafy greens such as spinach, dandelion greens, and kale, because these are blood thickeners. However, these veggies are a great source of nutrients, some of the best. So I recommend counteracting the blood thickening effect by upping your intake of olive oil, fish oil, and sesame seed, which are natural blood thinners. Please be sure to talk to your doctor about this.

3. Consume good bacteria. Your body needs healthy bacteria to help you digest your food and absorb all its nutrients. I recommend that my clients consume these bacteria daily. It is found naturally

in yogurt. If you're vegan or lactose intolerant, you can take an acidophilus supplement.

4. Eat whole grains. Avoid all white flour products such as white bread and regular pasta, but even keep your consumption of whole wheat low. Try to eat more brown rice, quinoa, millet, rye, and cornmeal instead.

5. Consume foods to get your circulatory system moving. Specifically, try to add more cayenne pepper, garlic, and parsley to your diet to help naturally reduce your blood pressure.

6. Avoid processed sugar and caffeine. Women these days are generally so stressed that we burn out our adrenal glands, which is terrible for our health. It throws our hormones out of balance and makes us feel exhausted all the time. The usual response to being tired is to consume caffeine and sugar, but the more you do, the worse it gets. You get a temporary rush, but then you come crashing down harder than ever. I advise that you avoid processed sugar and caffeine as much as possible, although it's okay to drink a cup or two of green each day.

• *Supplements*: You can't get all the nutrients you need from our over-farmed, over-depleted soil and foods that have been picked, processed, and shipped too much and too soon. So I recommend that you supplement your diet with these substances:

1. B complex vitamin. These are the anti-stress vitamins. They nourish the nervous system, help us manage stress and anxiety, and balance our hormones. They're like the electrical wiring in our bodies. Take at least one hundred milligrams per day of a B-complex supplement. You may also want to add a little extra B-12 in order to help your body turn the greens you consume into usable iron, and a folic acid supplement, which promotes heart health. B-6 acts as a natural diuretic, so try to avoid taking it if you're on medications that are diuretics. You should take these vitamins during the day.

2. Fatty acids (Omega 3, 6, and 9). If B-vitamins are the body's electrical wiring, then fatty acids are the insulation tape. The best kind of fatty acid for the heart is fish oil, with flaxseed oil as your second choice. I recommend trying to get your fish oil from wild-caught fresh fish, or frozen if you must. I advise against canned fish because these tend to absorb aluminum from the can. However, you can also take fish and flaxseed oil supplements if you don't want to eat fish. It's best to take these at night because we tend to burp them up. Freezing them first and taking them

with food will also help alleviate this unpleasant side effect.

3. Calcium. Calcium is the grounding cord for your nervous system. It's an emotional and structural support, and it's very important for the heart muscle. Magnesium works well with calcium to help relieve stress, so you can also take a calcium-magnesium supplement. Take these pills at bedtime to help promote good sleep.

4. Co-Q10. This enzyme helps keep your circulatory system stay in excellent working order. Take 50 to 200 milligrams per day depending on your state of health. Please consult with a health care specialist to determine how much is right for you.

5. Herbs to reduce cholesterol. Most women with heart disease have high cholesterol levels. To naturally bring your cholesterol levels down, consume plenty of dark, leafy greens and grapefruit, but also try these herbs: Chinese red rice yeast extract and Guggal lipids (from Ayurvedic medicine).

•   *Stress Management*: In addition to eating right and consuming the proper supplements, it's crucial to your overall health and wellness that you take care of your body by moving and breathing. I'm a big fan of yoga, which accomplishes both at the same time, and helps reduce stress. Some people enjoy doing cardio as well, which is great. You should exercise at least twenty minutes most days of the week. I also consider massage and deep bodywork a necessity, not a luxury.

HEART ON

Changing Your Life

According to a 2005 article in *Fast Company*, two years after undergoing coronary artery bypass surgery, ninety percent of people have *not* changed their lifestyles. Dr. Dean Ornish, however, seems to have come up with a method that works. In 1993, he ran a study (paid for by Mutual of Omaha) in which 333 patients with severely clogged arteries attended twice-weekly group support sessions led by a psychologist, got help quitting smoking, and took instruction in meditation, relaxation, yoga and aerobic exercise.

The program lasted just one year, but after three years, seventy-seven percent of the patients had stuck with their lifestyle changes and avoided further by-pass or angioplasty surgeries. It also saved Mutual of Omaha around $300,000 per patient.

Why did it work? Dr. Dean Ornish's program avoided using fear of death as a motivator, as is typically the case, but rather promises of a better life. He offered patients an inspired vision of "the joy of living." They talked about such pleasures as what it would be like to feel better, live longer, enjoy walking more, and making love again. "Joy is a more powerful motivator than fear," says Dr. Dean. Appealing to emotions works better than presenting people with a bunch of facts.

8.

WHEN LIFE GIVES
YOU LEMONS…

I postpone death by living, by suffering,
by error, by risking, by giving, by losing.

—ANAIS NIN

I never got an answer to my why.

No matter what I did, how much time I meditated and prayed, or experts I asked, the answer never came. No one could tell me why I got heart disease. The litany of unresolved questions circling around that question might have changed, but the core remained constant—an impenetrable mystery.

The Heart Truth

This year, four percent of women will be diagnosed with breast cancer. Forty-four percent will be diagnosed with heart disease.

It was to remain a mystery until my fifty-fifth birthday. That was the day my mom called to tell me she was in the hospital—having a heart attack. Sound familiar?

"What?" I asked in shock. "Where are you, really? Mom this isn't funny... Is Dad there? What's going on?" I felt my heart beating faster and faster with each "what."

She said, "I had the girls over for cards today. We had apple martinis and I told them it was your birthday so we all had a toast. Before I went to bed, I took my antibiotic, so at first I just thought I was having a bad reaction. Daddy told me to go back to sleep. But I knew something was wrong from the stories in your book. I got nauseous and my heart began to really race. I told Daddy to call the ambulance. When we got to the hospital, they checked me out. It was a heart attack, I was right—your book saved my life."

For once in my life I didn't want to be right, I didn't want to say, "I told you so." My face felt frozen. My ears were throbbing like I was sinking deeper and deeper underwater. And now my heart was thumping erratically, which is never good for me.

So many images passed before my eyes and across my chest: the moment when I first heard the words "heart attack" and my name in the same sentence, when they had me hooked up to monitors after the surgery, when I kept demanding "Why? Why me?" And now here it was again, the same old feeling, only it was *my mother*.

"Mom, are you sure? Did the doctors tell you *for sure* it was a heart attack?" Here I was diving head first into the family pool of denial.

"Pamela, I am laying on a bed all hooked up in an emergency room. Yes, I'm sure. And I'm scared."

"Don't be scared," I said, though I myself was petrified. "They know what they're doing and you are in a great heart hospital."

"They want to operate immediately."

"No way," I said.

"We need to get you a second opinion. Then we'll decide where how and who will do it." It was *déjà vu*, but now at least I could be in the driver's seat. My invincible mother, after all, was the original Energizer Bunny; she could put my energy in her back pocket. I couldn't imagine life without her.

In my own heart, my mother now became the wise one, the one I never fought with, the one who never opposed my choices in life or my lipstick color. That same woman who could drive me crazy over anything was now the woman I most admired and wanted to save.

My book galleys were still on my night table, and I saw the cover quote from Dr. Mehmet Oz as I drifted off. Dr. Oz is a heart surgeon who knows the heart inside and out. How ironic: there sat one of the leading heart surgeons in the country—not yet America's and Oprah's top doc, but a lifesaver, for sure—and his quote was on my book, even though we never met. I had no reserve in calling him about my mother, why not start with the best.

He answered his phone, "Mehmet here."

"Mehmet," I said. "You don't know me, but you gave me a quote for my book, and now my mother…"

"Come to see me tomorrow morning," he said. Wow serendipity strikes again. Watching this unfold for my mother was indeed grace personified.

We marched into his office the next day, the heart-clogged family en masse, the Cholesterol Express. I had been elevated to CEO status after my heart event. The nurse took our histories: me—triple bypass, Dad—valve replacement and stents; Mom—heart attack four days ago; my brother—shaking in his boots.

Dr. Oz explained what was happening in medical speak, he had his trademark calm and soulful exchange which set us all at ease. Collectively the family took a deep breath; and knew we were in the right hands. He gave my mother a choice of timing, getting her ready without the panic involved. "Wow, I never had that choice," He took her hands, held them, looked her in the eyes and said it would be a privilege to operate if she chose to do so. I'd had a surgeon leaning over me and telling me how dire my diagnosis was. He offered her meditation tapes to calm her down and a massage once she was done in the hospital program. I'd gotten a bedpan and a two-week hospital stay. He assured her of the success rates and informed her of any risks. She was immediately smitten, and wanted to sign up immediately.

"Why should I wait?" she blurted out. "I'm ready now."

We all got whiplash and told her to calm down. What nerve, for her to be so empowered by this. I had been a wuss, crying when they told me, crying like a baby as I made my will. This was a movie playing out, and finally my mother got the role she had been seeking for so long: the star of the show.

I sat with my mother for the following days, giving her all the information that I had culled about heart. It was sort of like her telling me the facts of life when I was a teenager, only less thrilling. I told her of the depression that followed the operation, the potential lack of sleep from the chest being cut open. I told her she would now feel her heart in a new way. I told her that she might have a lot of fear at first, but that she would learn how to communicate better with her energy. I told her this was the most performed operation, and that the doctors knew what they were doing. I even told her, "Who knows? Maybe Oprah is in your future." Of course that soothed her.

I tried to anticipate everything she would need when she awoke. I bought her a beautiful bed tray for when she came home, a back pillow to lean up against, creams to erase her scars, and a soft blanket to mess up with the goo from her wounds. I made her CDs of her favorite music, songs that would elevate her heart and her mood. I got her a slew of natural remedies that I had stumbled into during my recovery. I stocked her house with vitamins and healthy foods for soups and smoothies since her appetite would be low from the nausea and the meds. She used to hate it when I brought my healthy foods to her house, but now she couldn't stop me.

We waited a week to prepare her, the house, her brother and twin sister, countless friends, and, of course, my father. He needed as much time as possible. My father was getting increasingly agitated as the big day approached. This was, after all, his beloved Gloria. Married fifty-six years, they were never apart and still sweethearts. They danced together, got sick together, went to afternoon movies, and played cards together. Life would not exist for either one of them without the other. What would he possibly do without her? I could not think about that. I knew he never would admit any of this out loud, but I began to see him praying all the time as we got closer to the operation, prayer shawl and yarmulke in tow, relying on his faith to carry him, just as he had in my hospital room. He had even changed my name so death couldn't find me, an old religious custom.

The day of the operation was filled with serendipity.

As I got to the hospital, a messenger approached me with a big envelope. I was confused. Who knew I was there? I opened it to find the hardcover copy of my book, *Take it to Heart* with its red shiny cover, first one off the press from my publisher, Amy Hertz. Although my excitement was eclipsed by the moment at hand for my mother, I knew that this news would make her so happy.

She was all prepped waiting patiently with all of us surrounding her on the gurney, ready for combat, hair wrapped up in one of those hideous shower caps, wearing the prerequisite light blue hospital gown , tied in the back with a little bit of booty showing, sans makeup. This is not the Gloria any of us are used to seeing but she shined nonetheless. My mothers idea of being prepped was getting a mani-pedi and leg wax before the operation: Women will be women no matter the venue. My father was his humorous self, cracking jokes with the nurses, and trying to take charge of something. My brother Teddy was very serious; this heart business was all too much for him. Three out of four in the family down—was he next?

I showed my mother the book. She beamed with pride, and at that same moment Dr. Oz came over to take her away. His quote had made the cover, and there he was to wheel my mother off to another destiny. How could this man, whom I had never met, be on the cover of my story and now making another one for my mother in the same moment? Yes, still more questions.

We hovered around her for the send-off, planting our kisses and wishes as Dr. Oz whisked her away. My father began to tear up and took out his prayer book, which made me and Teddy cry.

I went inside myself to stay in visualization with her during the operation. I knew that the procedure would take five to six hours, so I needed to shore up. I was beginning to experience the feeling of fear that I had never gotten to feel for myself because I had always had to stay strong. I took deep breaths. My friend Carole brought us all lunch. My aunt and uncle were calling me every half hour. I took to roaming the halls. How did a hospital get to be so familiar to me? I knew where everything was. I knew I would be here for the days ahead.

About three hours in, I saw Dr. Oz walking towards us. My heart stopped: three hours was way too short. What had happened? How could it be? I couldn't read his face to tell if he was upset. I knew I was, I blurted out, "Is everything ok?"

Dr. Oz gave us his trademark big smile, "She's done. She did very well. She'll be up in an hour or so in ICU."

What? Three hours and she was done? Of course my mother could beat my record. Who else? Dr. Oz told us that he hadn't even needed to scar her leg, whereas I have a snake crawling up mine. He had only made a tiny incision on her chest, whereas mine was panoramic. Her heart surgery upstaged mine, she was seventy-seven and I was forty-seven? Was this really the conversation going on in my head?

Then I stopped myself... How could I be competing with my mother over *heart surgery*? Actually what I was really feeling was the differences in the last eight years surrounding the advances of heart surgery and women, and the gratitude I had that my mother was the recipient.

Needless to say, in the weeks and months that followed she began her own healing journey. Three months in, I did something that I hoped would help her speed up the healing process. I had gotten an offer to be on TV about my book, and I asked the producer if we could make the piece a "like daughter like mother" look into the role reversal caused of illness. I knew the thought of the cameras rolling would make her feel normal a bit faster than it might take normally. My bet paid off because the actress and fighter in her pulled it off beautifully. And the truth is, that's how it has been since then: my mother following in my heartbeats.

After my mother's heart attack and my own experience at the Mayo Clinic, where I was sent as part of the Womenheart's program to be a heart mentor, I was ready: Ready to serve others, ready to fully accept and embrace my heart disease on another level. I felt determined to make a difference in getting all the valuable information and my personal experience out into the neighborhoods, the doctor's offices, into the living rooms and offices, the yoga studios, and community forums where women would be sure to gather.

> ## The Heart Truth
> **For many women, the first symptom of heart disease is death.**

What remained with me most from my week at the Mayo Clinic were the other women's stories: horrifying, funny, poignant, and illuminating. And these, I knew, were just a handful of the stories that longed to be told. My thought was, imagine if we could create an open invitation to women everywhere to share their heart events? All those hearts filled like jelly donuts with life's lessons oozing out. What a magnificent troupe we could assemble.

Women remember everything about their heart events.

Their first one when their lives forever changed. What they were wearing. What they were thinking. What they were eating. Who they were with. What would be lost.

I knew I couldn't take on the project on alone. It would take more than a village to accomplish this, I would need a small continent of helpers to reach the 8 million who already had heart disease and the millions more that remained in the dark. This seemed a mission only a best friend would take on, so I turned to my long-time friend Carole Isenberg to see if I could enlist her support in pursuing this passion. Carole always had been interested in women's issues. She spent most of her celebrated career championing wonderful works in the arts, including the Academy Award-winning feature film, *The Color Purple*. From her movies, television projects, and workshops, she understood the issues women faced. It wasn't a hard sell; Carole jumped on the bandwagon immediately. But little did we know what we were getting ourselves into…

We knew that we wanted to create something unique to bring the attention of all women as well as doctors, the media, politicians, health care providers, and advocacy groups around the world to this crucial issue of heart disease among women. We knew that we wanted to use storytelling. We knew that we wanted the arts to be our platform and delivery system. And we knew that we needed recognizable names and faces to help bring this subject into the spotlight. We also needed to name it. After playing with endless permutations around the word "heart" and running the choices by our maven network of friends, we chose *Events of the Heart*.

Finally we decided to create a non-profit. Oy vey! Establishing a non-profit is not for anyone lacking in patience. You need to have a powerful vision and stamina to get your 501(c)3. You need to stay positive because there are endless roadblocks to this process. But we did get it, and so we began the business at heart.

Novartis Pharmaceuticals came aboard soon after with a grant, and their generous support helped birth Events of the Heart (EOH) into the world. A woman named Barbara Tombros embraced our vision and helped us make this a reality many women could benefit from. During this time, we continued to educate ourselves about women and heart disease so we could understand more about what was needed to make a difference. As we became clearer, we were able to articulate a mission statement, "Events of the Heart is a 501(c)3 non-profit organization dedicated to telling the real truth about women and heart disease. Using the creative arts and the media, EOH is building a community of women across America who understand the importance and power of a healthy heart." While we were at it, we made a wish list for our future.

We decided to introduce EOH on Monday October 2, 2007 at Jazz at Lincoln Center in New York City. What a night! It was a magical event. Writers from film and TV, poets and playwrights and journalists generously gave their time to write pieces, which actors dramatized that evening, bringing all things happening to the hearts of women to life. We called this special piece of theater *Heart On!* Joy Behar from *The View* was the mistress of ceremonies for a luminous cast of performers including Marcia Gay Harden, Holland Taylor, and Bob Balaban. My mother's very own renowned cardiovascular surgeon Dr. Mehmet Oz was honored with our first "You've Gotta Have Heart" award for his outstanding work communicating the reality of heart disease among women to the world.

I had the chance to bring my mother on stage and, as Oprah would say, gave her a full circle moment being up there with Dr. Oz and myself. My dear editor MeiMei Fox dubbed the event, "The Angina Monologues."

It was our plan to have this piece of theater travel around the country. Now that we had a template, we could refine our message. For our next venue, we headed out West to Los Angeles. On Monday, April 28, 2008, EOH opened at The Geffen Playhouse. For this smashing evening, the *Desperate Housewives* Eva Longoria, Dana Delany, and Brenda Strong left Wisteria Lane. Joining them were Holland Taylor, Jeffrey Tambor, Steven Collins, and Judy Gold, along with a group of other talented actors.

What we learned from these performances was a major lesson. Women were listening and they were responding, both to the emotional content and the facts. They came up to us after the shows and told us how deeply they had been affected. They said that they wanted to help—to talk about their own heart disease experiences and to become advocates.

We have only just begun our journey with Events of the Heart. There are many steps still yet to take. What we have learned is that we are reaching women through the stories of other women. Somehow in the intimacy, raw emotionality, and eloquence of these theatrical pieces, women could finally hear the message: "This could be you! It is *likely* to be you or someone very close to you." They grasped the importance. We finally had a home in women's hearts.

A decade has passed since my heart events and I am fifty-seven years old now. Getting here has taken every part of me: the part that grew me up, the part that put me back together again, and the part that opened my heart to my life. Heart disease has become the greatest teacher of my life. My heart was always the biggest and strongest part of me, even though it seems it was also the most vulnerable. Today those two facts are integrated, not separated. And for the most part I am re-enchanted with life, though of course I still have heart OFF days as we all do. In spite of the minor ailments, I would not trade a day of all these experiences for anything else. These heartbeats were and are the way I stay on course with myself.

So what's life like now? Well lets start with first things first. I eat what I love, I have an occasional drink, and I even have that ice cream cone now and then. I taste experiences with the right balance of caution and abandon, and I am guided by the fact that each and every moment is the only one I have. I continually invite God into steering my life, knowing that everything is uncertainty but faith.

I realized after all was said and done that all I ever really wanted to do in all my many careers was to spread *heart*. Heart disease has given me the chance to do just that. Here the opportunity all along was, ticking inside me, right at the center of my being.

♡ *You never know where the YES will turn up amidst the ocean of no's.*

Since talking is one of the things women do best, let's use our voices—our deep passionate voices—to break the silence, crack the code, and come into conversation about why heart disease is claiming the lives of so many American women. We deserve more thorough medical research, better equipment, proper diagnosis and improved treatment—and we need to demand it. Do you realize how powerful *you* really are? Behind the picket fences and wisteria hedges in houses, at work at home and in offices, giving presentations in boardrooms, women take everything to heart and are at the heart of everything. Did you know that we're responsible for eighty percent of all consumer purchases? We could change heart disease policies in this country with a one-day shopping boycott! That would get some attention, don't you think?

Let's do it. Let's make heart disease our juiciest gossip, our best-selling cover story, our hottest new tip. Let's take it on and not let go until we can walk all together, open hearted. Yes, it's true, we women truly have always been the real heart *on* for each other.

HEALING THE HEART

Use Your Voice

By Dr. Suzanne Steinbaum, Director of Women and Heart Disease, Lenox Hill Hospital

As a cardiologist whose specialty is women and heart disease, I often see women who have made multiple visits to many different doctors and whose complaints have been written off as "anxiety," "stress," or just something "in your head." By the time they reach my office, these women are frustrated and scared, because in their hearts they know that there is something is truly wrong with their hearts. It is true the heart disease often presents itself differently in women than in men, and is more difficult to diagnose. Their symptoms are often so obscure that sometimes having a heart condition might be the last guess of even educated medical professionals.

With heart disease being the number one killer of women, and still the most under-diagnosed and often mistreated illness, women need to empower themselves. Pamela's story is real and true. It serves as a powerful reminder of how difficult it is to not only become ill, but also to become a number and a statistic. A typical woman heart disease patient has to battle not only herself, but also the medical community in having her heart properly cared for.

Women need to understand that they can fight this disease and win the battle. They need to know their risks, as early in life as they can, and pay attention to them. Unfortunately, we are not invincible. Yet we are given choices and we are given our genes.

If we know both intimately, we can get information that will make us stronger and help us become empowered. No one really needs to get sick from heart disease. Each person simply has to learn the best way to live the fight against it. Pamela's story is one that I tell over and over again. I hope it can serve as a rallying cry for us all.

Top Twenty-Four Heart Ons and Heart Offs

A heart *on* is an act that makes the heart feel alive, a feeling that enters right through the soul. Heart *offs* and heart attacks are the ways your heart and soul tell you that you are in need of attention and balance.

Here are my personal heart *ons*, the ones that I live by now:

1. Putting myself first by saying no to that which doesn't serve me (this is the hardest one for women, by the way).
2. Getting out of my head and learning to find the answers from my heart.
3. Taking time for pleasure, passion, and creativity so that I can be versed in the language of my heart's desires.
4. Not waiting for anyone else to fulfill my heart's desire.
5. Being grateful for everything in my life.
6. Acknowledging my heart for the incredible journey it has taken me on.

7. Allowing myself and others to be as they are, without judging, blaming, or fixing.
8. Accepting the journey as *right*, just the way it is.
9. Eating with love, as though food were my greatest healer.
10. Moving my body—dance, walk, stretch, make love—so that my heart can breathe.
11. Getting things off my chest in real time.
12. Express what I feel without reacting to it.

My **Heart *Offs***, the things I avoid:

1. Overdoing it.
2. Being reactive through eating, drinking, shopping, or otherwise abusing myself.
3. Not following my inner voice.
4. Being in places or with people that don't make me feel alive.
5. Being in toxic relationships with people who cannot meet me in a heartfelt dialogue.
6. Too much noise, the kind inside my head and outside my life.
7. Winters in New York City.
8. Traveling down the dark Road of Regrets.
9. Being told what is best for me by someone else.
10. Going too fast for too long without a break.
11. Forgetting it's the process that matters, not the destination.
12. Not taking responsibility for my choices.

STRAIGHT
FROM THE HEART

Resources for Women with Heart Disease

Heart-Disease Related Organizations

Events of the Heart

www.eventsoftheheart.org

Events of the Heart is a 501(c)3 non-profit organization dedicated to telling the real truth about women and heart disease. Using the creative arts and the media, EOH is building a community of women across America who understand the importance and power of a healthy heart. Through books, workshops, videos, theater, and film, Events of the Heart's mission is to educate women about every aspect of heart disease—from prevention to genetic factors to the emotional and physical facets of the recovery process—and to empower women to live heart healthy. Come and see the true stories in *Dear Heart* adapted for the stage and performed by well-known celebrities at the next Events of the Heart production.

WomenHeart
www.womenheart.org

WomenHeart is the only national patient-centered organization that provides support, education and advocacy for women living with heart disease. Through a coalition of national volunteers and community-based support networks, online support services, and educational programs, WomenHeart offers comprehensive services to women with heart disease and those at-risk, and empowers all women to take charge of their heart health.

Sister to Sister
www.sistertosister.org

Sister to Sister: Everyone Has a Heart Foundation, Inc., is a 501(c)3 non-profit organization dedicated exclusively to the *prevention* of heart disease in women. Their sponsors enable them to provide free cholesterol screenings to women around the country. Sister to Sister does not provide any treatment-related information nor do they recommend or endorse any products. Sister to Sister is not a patient advocacy organization.

American Heart Association

www.goredforwomen.org

The American Heart Association is a national voluntary health agency whose mission is: "Building healthier lives, free of cardiovascular diseases and stroke." The AHA's *Go Red For Women* campaign celebrates the energy, passion and power we have as women to band together to wipe out heart disease and stroke. Thanks to the participation of millions of people across the country, the color red and the red dress now stand for the ability all women have to improve their heart health and live stronger, longer lives. Today, the near-term goal is nothing less than a 25% reduction in coronary heart disease and stroke risk by the year 2010.

National Heart Lung and Blood Institute

www.nhlbi.nih.gov/health/hearttruth/

The NHLBI plans, conducts, fosters, and supports an integrated and coordinated program of basic research, clinical investigations and trials, observational studies, and demonstration and education projects. To make women more aware of the danger of heart disease, the NHLBI and partner organizations are sponsoring a national campaign called *The Heart Truth*. The campaign's goal is to give women a personal and urgent wake-up call about their risk of heart disease. The centerpiece of *The Heart Truth* is the Red Dress, which was introduced as the national symbol for women and heart disease awareness in

2002 by NHLBI. The Red Dress reminds women of the need to protect their heart health, and inspires them to take action.

Heart Healthy Women
www.hearthealthywomen.org

The mission at Heart Healthy Women is to provide women with in-depth, up-to-date information on the prevention, diagnosis, and treatment of heart and blood vessel diseases, eliminate gender and racial disparities in the diagnosis and treatment of cardiovascular disease, and increase the participation of women in clinical trials of cardiovascular disease.

MY FAVORITE HEART HEALERS

Dr. Jane-Iris Farhi
Cardiologist, Private Practice
1075 Park Avenue
New York, NY 10128
(212) 722-0854

Dr. Suzanne Steinbaum
Director, Women and Heart Disease, Heart and Vascular
    Institute
Attending Cardiologist, Lenox Hill Hospital
130 East 77th Street, 9th Floor
New York, New York 10021
(212) 434-6902

(212) 434-2606
www.srsheart.com
www.forwomenshearts.com

Dr. Mehmet Oz
Professor of Surgery, Columbia University Medical Center
Director, Cardiovascular Institute, Columbia University
        Medical Center
Vice Chairman, Cardiovascular Services, Department of Surgery
New York Presbyterian Hospital
(212) 305-4434

Dr. Michael Roizen
Institute Chair, Chief Wellness Officer, Wellness Institute,
        Cleveland Clinic
Cardiothoracic Anesthesiologist
Cleveland Clinic Main Campus
Mail Code TR2-01
9500 Euclid Avenue
Cleveland, OH 44195
(216) 444-2595

Dr. Gregory Costa
Chiropractor, Homeopathy, Private Practice
698 West End Avenue, Apt. 1A
New York, NY 10025
(212) 864-6127

Oz Garcia, Ph.D.
Celebrity Nutritionist and Executive Chairman, OZ
    Wellness Corporation
10 West 74th Street
New York, NY 10023
www.ozgarcia.com

Oonaja Malagon
Yoga, Qigong, Energy healing
(845) 657-6280

New York Dermatology Group
David Colbert
119 Fifth Ave, 4th Floor
New York NY 10003
(212) 533-8888
www.davidcolbertmd.com

Dr. Doris Day
General, Cosmetic, Laser, and Surgical Dermatology,
    Private Practice
135 East 71st Street
New York, NY 10021
(212) 772-0740
www.myclearskin.com

Sally Kravich
The Natural Health Expert
M.S. Holistic Nutrition, C.N.H.P., Consultant, Iridologist
New York: (212) 946-1623
Los Angeles: (310) 285-3528
www.sallykravich.com

Dr. Frank Lipman
Integrative Medicine, Homeopathy, General Practitioner
Founder and Director, Eleven Eleven Wellness Center
32 West 22nd St, 5th Floor
New York, NY 10010
(212) 255-1800
www.lipmanworld.com

Pamela Miles
Reiki Healer, Integrative Medicine Specialist
www.ReikiInMedicine.org

MeiMei Fox
Life Coach, Yoga Teacher, Writer
San Francisco, CA
www.meimeifox.com

Scott Berliner
Specializes in integrative approaches to health care through
supplementation and good diet.

Life Science Pharmacy
144 Route 17M, Suite #4
Harriman, NY 10926
(845) 781-7613
www.lifesciencepharmacy.com

Dr. Gerald Curatola
Rejuvenation Dentistry
521 Park Avenue
New York, New York 10065
(212) 355-4777
www.rejuvenationdentistry.com

DIAGNOSTIC TEST:

According to several doctors interviewed for this book, the Ultrafast CT scan is probably the best diagnostic test for heart disease. If your health insurance does not want to pay for the test, you might consider paying for it yourself. Call 800-NEW-TEST.

SHOP FOR THE CAUSE:

The Sweetheart Bracelet
http://www.eventsoftheheart.org/product_center.asp
The symbol of *Take it to Heart!* Designed by yours truly, author Pamela Serure. Give it to all the sweethearts in your life: mothers, wives, daughters, best friends, and of course, yourself.

Books to Recover By:

Essential Rumi, by Coleman Barks. A Rumi poem a day keeps the blues away.

Letters to a Young Poet, by Rainer Maria Rilke, translated by Stephen Mitchell. I reread this piece every year, especially number eight.

Love in the Second Act: True Stories of Romance, Midlife and Beyond by Alison Leslie Gold. Nothing heals the heart like a good love story.

God in All Worlds: An Anthology of Contemporary Spiritual Writings, edited by Lucinda Vardey.

Cries of the Spirit, edited by Marilyn Sewell. The best compilation of poetry (my favorite is "Wild Geese" by Mary Oliver).

The Light Inside the Dark, by John Tarrant Harper. Definitely a light inside the dark tunnel of recovery.

You, the series by Mehmet C. Oz, M.D. and Michael F. Roizen, M.D.

One Thousand Days in Venice, by Marlena de Blasi and *One Thousand Days in Tuscany*, by Marlena de Blasi. If anything can take you out of yourself it's a foodie /travel love story. These are fantastic.

Any of Ruth Reichl's or MFK Fisher's books, they are masters of memoir and food and balms to women recovery process.

Twenty Love Poems and a Song of Despair, by Pablo Neruda. With a glass of red wine, this is a perfect date.

The Soulmate Secret, by Arielle Ford. She found hers with this method and invites you to do the same.

Start Where you Are: A Guide to Compassionate Living, by Pema Chodron. She always guides you gently back to your self.

The Prophet, by Khalil Gibran. Wisdom no matter what age or time of your life.

Meetings With Remarkable Men, by G I Gurdjieff. When your soul needs a good teaching this is the book to read.

My iPod Playlist to Recover By:

Ok, this is my favorite all-time anthem.
I guess because so much change did come.
Pick an artist you love and play it over and over.

- "A Change Is Gonna Come," Leela James
- "A Change Is Gonna Come," Seal
- "A Change Is Gonna Come," Bobby Womack
- "A Change Is Gonna Come," Aaron Neville
- "A Change Is Gonna Come," Tina Turner
- "A Change Is Gonna Come," Sam Cooke
- "A Change Is Gonna Come," Aretha Franklin
         …you get the idea.
- "Crying," k.d. lang
- "Calling All Angels," Jane Siberry with k.d. lang
- "If I Could Turn Back the Hands of Time," R. Kelly
- "The Way I Am," Ingrid Michaelson
- "Anyone Who Had a Heart," Shelby Lynne
- "In My Secret Life," by Leonard Cohen
- "Don't Leave Me This Way," Thelma Houston
- "Stand By Me," Seal
- "Stand By Me," John Lennon
- "Hallelujah," k.d. lang
- "It's a Man's Man's Man's World," Seal
- "Make You Feel My Love," Adele
- "You Don't Have to Say You Love Me," Shelby Lynne
- "How Can I Be Sure," Shelby Lynne

- "I've Been Loving You Too Long," Seal
- "I (Who Have Nothing)," Ben E. King
- "Summertime," Billy Stewart
- "It Ain't Me, Babe," Bob Dylan
- "The Quest," Bryn Christopher
- "I Have Nothing/I Will Always Love You," Charice
- "I'm Still In Love With You," Seal
- "Viva la Vida," Coldplay
- "Don't Leave Me This Way," Harold Melvin & The Blue Notes
- "Unchained Melody," Righteous Brothers
- "Everybody Knows," Rufus Wainwright
- "I'm Your Man," Nick Cave
- "I'd Do Anything for Love (But I Won't Do That)," Meat Loaf
- "Tell Him," Lauryn Hill
- "(Sittin' On)," Sara Bareilles
- "Anniversary Song," Eva Cassidy
- "Never Can Say Goodbye," Isaac Hayes
- "Brothers & Sisters," Bongmaster Inc
- "Love Is A Losing Game," Amy Winehouse
- "This Is My Life," Shirley Bassey
- "Ooh Child (Alternate Version)," Beth Orton
- "The Closest Thing To Crazy," Katie Melua
- "Sally Go Round The Roses," Damnations
- "Misty Blue," Dorothy Moore
- "I Who Have Nothing," Shirley Bassey
- "Feeling Good," Nina Simone
- "No One," Alicia Keys

My Favorite Healing Quotes:

I have never met a person whose greatest need was anything other than real, unconditional love. You can find it in a simple act of kindness toward someone who needs help. There is no mistaking love. You feel it in your heart. It is the common fiber of life, the flame that heals our soul, energizes our spirit, and supplies passion to our lives. It is our connection to God and to each other.

—Elizabeth Kubler-Ross

I ache in the places I used to to play.

—Leonard Cohen

The greatest weakness of most humans is their hesitancy to tell others how much they love them while they're alive.

—Unknown

God always answers in the deeps, never in the shallows of our soul.

—Unknown

Everyone should carefully observe which way his heart draws him, and then choose that way with all his strength.

—Hasidic saying

Who looks outside, dreams. Who looks inside, awakens.

—Carl Jung

To understand the heart and mind of a person, look not at what he has already achieved, but at what he aspires to.

—KHALIL GIBRAN

You will find as you look back upon your life that the moments when you have truly lived are the moments when you have done things in the spirit of love.

—HENRY DRUMMOND

I am the feminine qualities: fame, beauty, perfect speech, memory, intelligence, loyalty, and forgiveness.

—THE BHAGAVAD GITA

Oh darling, let your body in, let it tie you in comfort.

—ANNE SEXTON

I am running into a new year
And the old years blow back, like a wind
That catch my hair
Like strong hair, like all my old promises
And it will be hard to let go
Of what I said to myself, and about myself
When I was sixteen, twenty-six, thirty-six
Even thirty-six but
I am running into a new year
And I beg what I love and leave to forgive me

—LUCILLE CLIFTON

For one human being to love another; that is perhaps the most difficult of all our tasks, the ultimate, the last test and proof, the work for which all other work is but preparation.

—Rainer Maria Rilke

Look for a long time at what pleases you, and a longer time at what pains you.

—Collette

One is not born a woman, but becomes one.

—Simone de Beauvoir

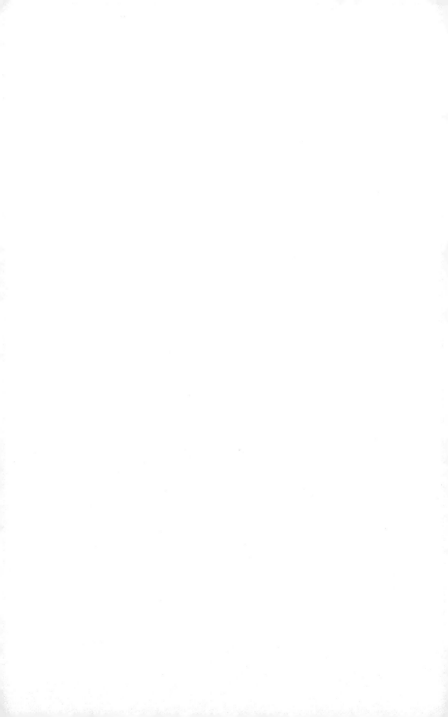

ACKNOWLEDGMENTS

I have so much to be grateful for and to. This book is only a partial reflection of all that has happened to me since my bypass, a small token of the grace that has been bestowed upon me. It is so clear to me now that we can never recover and renew alone; it does take a village, a city and a universe sometimes. Upon this winding path, not only do you encounter challenges but also angels like-minded souls and many acts of random kindnesses. Some people have always been there; some were brand new like my new life, and some just fit in as if they were a missing piece. All of them make my heart better and better because of who they are.

Mom and Dad, thank you for being exactly who you are and

loving me for who I am. I counted on you and you delivered time and time again. My Carola, day-by-day you inspire me to slow down, use my heart with love and compassion, and remind me that there is more time for all the things I want to do. Dr. Jesse Hanley, you are a true healer and inspiration for women and their hearts, thank you for healing mine. Dr. Jane Farhi, you ushered me to safety with my heart time and again. Dr. Suzanne Steinbaum, you follow your heart while taking care of so many others. Dr. Mehmet Oz, your heart and soul know no bounds.

To all my friends who helped me climb back up on the horse and made my ride easier… Geneen, thank you for those loving cups of tea and bowls of soup, and for taking charge of everything with heart. To KT, who made me remember my adventures weren't over yet. To Donna Karan for making my recovery look and feel so beautiful. To Mo, who bought me my first Mac and told me to write my story. To Raymond and Marlette for making California one big family for me. To Arielle Ford, who inspires and uplifts with her heart. To Debby Ford for chasing the shadows away. To Brian for his heart tunes. To Rabbi Judith, who through her prayers and teachings showed me grace. Sybil, thank you for bringing me back to my skills and laughing with me while climbing that mountain. To Denise and Tim for my magical 50th birthday. To Rosie for her wise counsel when I needed it most. To Josh, Lenore, Pavi, and GiGi, thanks for voting me into the family. To Zack and Lizzy for your love of family and sense of humor . To Bryan Bantry for mentoring me into producing great works. To peggy Siegal for opening her Rolodex

To my WomenHeart group, your lunches and friendship were essential to my diet

A heartfelt thanks to Laura Yorke, my agent who with her laser-sharp wit and precision made my story a book. To MeiMei Fox, a brilliant editor who walked more miles in my words than I thought possible. To Amy Hertz, who had the vision to know my story belonged to every woman.

To my Events of the Heart staff: Jessica, Erin, and Maria you have toiled and tilled the soil and brought up roses. To Marc Haeringer, who midwifed the new version of *Dear Heart*. To Barbara Tombrose for believing and allowing Events of the Heart to be born. To Brenda Strong, who is so wise and generous with her own heart on our behalf. To Benito: you drive me nuts but you drive me safely. To my brother, Teddy, my nieces, Gloria, Patti. and nephew Hymie and their new families. I hope you all learn from this family legacy. To all the actors in the creative communities who generously lent their voices, gave their time and their names for us to get noticed, GOD BLESS YOU!

To my Sage in heaven, I know you watch over me everyday.

To my Habebe, the extraordinary shih tzu who knows me, loves me, and licks me know matter what I do: your unconditional love has truly healed my heart.

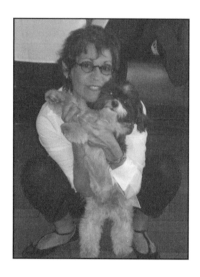

Pamela Serure, a respected health expert, lecturer, and the author of several books, has devoted her life to getting the word out about women and wellness. She is the co-founder and executive director of Events of the Heart, a non-profit organization dedicated to using the arts to raise awareness among women about heart disease. Prior to founding Events of the Heart, Serure developed the concept Get Juiced, as well as other products, and consulted with over 2,000 clients on how to achieve health and balance in their lives and business.

Serure is a red wine-loving, dark chocolate-eating foodie who has yet to meet a loaf of bread she didn't like. She is a native New Yorker, but escapes to sunny destinations every chance she gets.

For more information, please visit: *www.eventsoftheheart.org*.